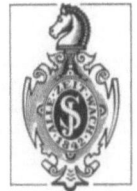

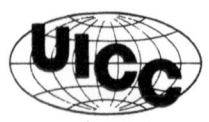 International Union Against Cancer

Treatment and Rehabilitation Programme

Chairman: Ismail Elsebai

Project on Current Treatment of Cancer

Ismail Elsebai, Chairman

H. Julian G. Bloom · Ian Burn · Folke Edsmyr † · Roberto A. Estevez
Joseph Fortner · Barth Hoogstraten

Coordinating Editor of this volume: Barth Hoogstraten

The series *Current Treatment of Cancer* consists of the following volumes:

Cancer in Children, 2nd edition (1986)

Hematologic Malignancies (1986)

Lung Tumors

Breast Cancer

Gynecological Tumours

Urogenital Tumours

Cancer of the Digestive Tract

Skin, Soft Tissue and Bone Tumours

Head and Neck Tumours

Tumours of the Nervous System

General Principles of Oncology

Hematologic Malignancies

Edited by B. Hoogstraten

With Contributions by
J. R. Durant   F. W. Gunz   E. S. Henderson   B. Hoogstraten
H. J. Iland   J. Laszlo   C. S. Portlock

With 10 Figures

Springer-Verlag Berlin Heidelberg New York
London Paris Tokyo

UICC, Rue du Conseil-Général 3, CH-1205 Geneva

Editor:

Dr. Barth Hoogstraten

Medical Director Cancer Treatment Center
Bethesda Hospital, Inc.
629 Oak Street, Suite 409
Cincinnati, OH 45206, USA

ISBN-13:978-3-540-16293-3   e-ISBN-13: 978-3-642-82734-1
DOI: 10.1007/978-3-642-82734-1

2121/3140-5 4 3 2 1 0

Members of the Project Current Treatment of Cancer

H. Julian G. Bloom
The Royal Marsden Hospital
Department of Radiotherapy
and Oncology
Downs Road
GB-Sutton, Surrey SM2 5PT
England

Ian Burn
British Association
of Surgical Oncology
Charing Cross Hospital
Fulham Palace Road
GB-London W6 8RF
England

Folke Edsmyr †
Department of Urological Oncology
Karolinska Sjukhuset
Radiumhemmet
P.O. Box 60500
S-10401 Stockholm
Sweden

Ismail Elsebai
National Cancer Institute Cairo
Kasr El-Aini Street
Cairo, Egypt

Roberto A. Estevez
Facultad de Medicina del Salvador
Catedra de Oncologia Clinica
Avenida Santa Fé 5089 9–20
1425 Buenos Aires, Argentina

Joseph Fortner
Memorial Sloan-Kettering
Cancer Center
York Avenue 1275
New York, NY 10021, USA

Barth Hoogstraten
Cancer Treatment Center
Bethesda Hospital, Inc.
629 Oak Street, Suite 409
Cincinnati, OH 45206, USA

Foreword

This new series on the treatment of cancer is sponsored by the UICC. The editors and authors feel strongly that more standardization is needed on a worldwide basis in cancer therapy. This, of course, is only possible if experts from all countries subscribe to a joint policy of making their treatment designs available to practising oncologists all over the world.

Current Treatment of Cancer will discuss all the equipment and methods now in use in cancer therapy. It will cover all types of cancer, thus providing the reader with comprehensive information on cancer management.

In recent decades there has been a tremendous improvement in the treatment of cancer, and there is hope for even further success in this fight. We are convinced that this series will help us to make a concerted response to the challenge of cancer.

UICC
Treatment and Rehabilitation Programme

Ismail Elsebai
Chairman

Preface

During the past two decades we have witnessed an exciting evolution in the understanding and management of hematologic malignancies. The number of drugs available 20 years ago for the treatment of acute leukemia was so small that the disease in children and in adults could be discussed within one chapter. Since then, rapid progress has been made in the management of childhood leukemia, making for a much better prognosis. Over the past 10 years we have seen the same developments in respect of leukemia in adults.

Great strides have been made in the histopathology of lymphoma. No longer is one name sufficient to cover the disease. Hodgkin's disease is clearly a separate entity and, unfortunately, we can do no better than use the term non-Hodgkin's lymphoma when discussing lymphomas of other histology. Hodgkin's disease, regarded as invariably fatal in the 1940s, is now curable in a large percentage of patients. We all owe a great debt of gratitude to Dr. Henry S. Kaplan, whose concepts of the fundamental nature and natural history of Hodgkin's disease led to better therapy. His contributions to the development of the linear accelerator have influenced the outcome of many forms of cancer. It was typical of the man to accept immediately when I invited him to write the chapter on Hodgkin's disease. He began, but could not finish.

Hematologists have been less successful in improving the outcome of chronic leukemias, myeloproliferative diseases, and multiple myeloma. Patience and tempered enthusiasm are often the best management of these diseases. The limited increase in survival that can be achieved does not always justify the side effects and cost of the drugs.

In this volume, the authors have each provided an authoritative treatise on their assigned topic. Each was given the freedom to express their thoughts about disease management and, where appropriate, to indicate how the disease is treated in their institution. No attempt was made to provide an in-depth review of the literature. I am grateful to the authors for prompt submission of their contributions, especially to Dr. John R. Durant, who at short notice so graciously substituted for Dr. Kaplan.

I am grateful to Bethesda Hospitals, Inc. for its cooperation during the preparation of this volume. Special thanks are due to Mrs. Shirley Viner, who participated in the entire editorial process and devoted many hours of labor to finalizing the manuscript.

Barth Hoogstraten

Contents

5. Non-Hodgkin's Lymphoma

C. S. Portlock

6. Multiple Myeloma

B. Hoogstraten

Contributors

John R. Durant, MD, FACP

President, Fox Chase Cancer Center
Philadelphia, PA 19111, USA

Frederick W. Gunz, MD, PhD

Formerly Director of Medical Research
Kanematsu Memorial Institute
Sydney Hospital, Sydney, Australia

Edward S. Henderson, MD

Chief of Medical Oncology
Roswell Park Memorial Institute
666 Elm Street
Buffalo, NY 14263, USA

Barth Hoogstraten, MD, FACP

Medical Director Cancer Treatment Center
Bethesda Hospital, Inc.
629 Oak Street, Suite 409
Cincinnati, OH 45206, USA

Harry J. Iland, MB, FRACP, FRCPA

Clinical Hematologist
Royal Prince Alfred Hospital
Camperdown, NSW 2050, Australia

John Laszlo, MD

Vice President for Research
American Cancer Society, Inc.
90 Park Avenue
New York, NY 10016, USA

Carol S. Portlock, MD

Yale University School of Medicine
Section of Medical Oncology
333 Cedar Street
New Haven, CT 06510, USA

1. Treatment of Chronic Leukemias

F. W. Gunz

Introduction

Chronic leukemias occur worldwide. There are two types—chronic myeloid (CML) or granulocytic and chronic lymphocytic (CLL). Their symptoms and physical signs differ from each other to some extent, as does their treatment. For this reason they will be described separately. Both types of chronic leukemia are rarer than the acute leukemias. In Western and many other populations CLL is more common than CML, but in Japan and elsewhere in the Far East CLL is very rarely encountered. The reason for this is unknown. CLL is a disease of late middle and old age and is never found in children. At least twice as many men as women have CLL. CML occurs occasionally in children and becomes more common as ages increase. This type is found slightly more often in males than in females.

The symptoms of both types of chronic leukemia are variable. Some patients, especially with CLL, have only mild or no symptoms for periods which may last many years. Others suffer a variety of symptoms from moderate to very severe. Neither type of chronic leukemia is curable by any agent now available, although symptoms can often be relieved and life sometimes prolonged by appropriate treatment. These facts should be borne in mind when the question of therapy is being considered: since no cure can be expected, only sufficient treatment should be planned to restore and maintain the patient's usual state of health, if indeed that is possible. There is no advantage in giving more than is needed for the control of symptoms, and excessive treatment may in fact be dangerous. As will be seen below, the management of chronic leukemia is often simple, especially in the early stages, but it may demand great skill and experience in patients with advanced disease.

Chronic Myeloid Leukemia

Clinical Picture

Occasionally CML is found accidentally in asymptomatic patients when blood counts are done for reasons unconnected with the disease. In most patients, however, CML causes symptoms, and the patient seeks help for this reason. Among the commonest symptoms are the following:

1. General ill health, often the result of anemia. There is pallor, weariness, and, with severe anemia, shortness of breath on exertion. Sometimes there is fever.
2. Abdominal distension, with or without the sensation of an actual tumor. This is caused by the enlarged spleen, which may be visible. Splenomegaly often gives rise to discomfort described as a "dragging" feeling, or to actual pain which can be severe, especially on inspiration. In such cases the spleen may be infarcted and the pain due to perisplenitis. Loss of appetite, or inability to eat more than small meals may result from pressure on the stomach by a grossly enlarged spleen. The liver is usually enlarged also.
3. Bleeding from the rectum or vagina, epistaxis, hematuria or hematemesis, or apparently spontaneous bruising, all associated with changes in platelet numbers or function or in the clotting factors.

Less common manifestations of CML include lymphadenopathy, pain and tenderness over the sternum or other bones, gout, and the symptoms of urinary calculi. Peptic — especially duodenal — ulceration not infrequently accompanies CML.

Laboratory Investigations

The symptomatology of CML, especially the often gross degree of hepatosplenomegaly, may be sufficiently characteristic to raise a strong suspicion of the diagnosis. Alternatively the symptoms can be more vague and puzzling. In either case a definitive diagnosis is impossible without appropriate laboratory tests, of which a blood count is by far the most important. Table 1 shows a typical blood count in CML.

The combination of a neutrophil leukocytosis higher than 50×10^9/liter with the presence of significant numbers of immature forms such as myelocytes and metamyelocytes, and associated with mild to moderate degrees of normocytic normochromic anemia and perhaps a raised platelet count, is sufficiently characteristic to make further diagnostic laboratory investigations unnecessary in many patients suspected of having CML. This is so particularly when such blood counts are seen together with typical clinical findings such as hepatosplenomegaly.

Table 1. Typical blood count in CML

Hemoglobin		125 g/liter
Erythrocytes		4.2×10^{12}/liter
Leukocytes		250×10^9/liter
Differential		
Neutrophils	60%	150×10^9/liter
Metamyelocytes	14%	35×10^9/liter
Myelocytes	12%	30×10^9/liter
Promyelocytes	1%	2.5×10^9/liter
Blasts	1%	2.5×10^9/liter
Basophils	4%	10×10^9/liter
Eosinophils	2%	5×10^9/liter
Lymphocytes	2%	5×10^9/liter
Monocytes	4%	10×10^9/liter
Platelets		600×10^9/liter
Reticulocytes		1%

Table 2. Further laboratory tests in CML

Test	CML	Normal
Bone marrow	Hyperplasia ++ M : E ratio 30 : 1 Megakaryocytes ++	Normal cellularity M : E ratio 3 : 1 Megakaryocytes +
Cytochemistry	Alkaline phosphatase score 0–5 per 100 leukocytes	Alkaline phosphatase score 15–75 per 100 leukocytes
Cytogenetics	Translocation 9 : 22 (Philadelphia chromosome)	Normal karyotype

When the blood count is less typical, further tests may need to be done. Thus the leukocyte count may be only moderately raised, there may be either few immature myeloid cells or substantial numbers of blasts or other primitive cells. Other unusual blood findings in CML are severe degrees of anemia or significant thrombocytopenia on presentation. In such cases it is probably obvious that the patient has a serious blood disease, but a specific diagnosis is required before the correct treatment can be begun. Alternative diagnoses, such as acute leukemia, myelofibrosis, or carcinomatosis with skeletal metastases must be excluded, and for this purpose additional investigations are essential. The most important of these are:

1. Bone marrow aspiration and, if possible, bone marrow biopsy

2. Blood cytochemistry, especially the leukocyte alkaline phosphatase score

3. Cytogenetic studies of blood and/or marrow

Table 2 shows the findings to be expected.

The discovery of a grossly hyperplastic bone marrow with heavy predominance of the myeloid cell series, and the presence of a very low leukocyte alkaline phosphatase score, make the diagnosis of CML virtually certain; the finding of Philadelphia chromosomes puts it beyond doubt. About 10% of cases with clinical and hematologic signs suggesting CML do not have the Philadelphia chromosome. These patients have an atypical disease which responds poorly to treatment and is probably not CML.

Management

Principles

Treatment for CML is given with the aims of relieving its symptoms and of maintaining the patient's health close to its normal state for as long as possible. The usual means of achieving this aim is through the use of chemotherapy. A single drug is generally employed, that preferred by most physicians being busulfan (Myleran). Ancillary drugs, especially allupurinol, are frequently required.

If treatment is successful, a characteristic train of events will be observed over the next 3 or 4 months: symptoms like lassitude, shortness of breath, abdominal distension or bleeding will diminish in severity and later disappear; the enlarged liver and spleen will shrink and may become impalpable; and blood counts will indicate a rising hemoglobin concentration, falling numbers of leukocytes and platelets, and the disappearance from the blood of immature and abnormal myeloid cells. Entirely normal blood counts can often be achieved. Similarly the composition of the bone marrow may change with a reduction in cellularity, an increase in the proportion of erythroid cells, and diminution in that of myeloid precursor cells. The neutrophil alkaline phosphate score often rises, but Philadelphia chromosomes do not disappear from the marrow, although they are no longer found in the blood. Their persistence in the marrow indicates persistence of the underlying leukemic process, despite the clinical impression that remission of the disease is complete. Eventual relapse must therefore be anticipated, although this can often be controlled by further therapy. A critical event in CML is the transition to a refractory phase which occurs in nearly all cases. It has been given many names, including those of blast crisis, acute transformation, and metamorphosis. Its management is extremely difficult since blast crisis, in the great majority of instances, is entirely refractory to all forms of therapy.

Chemotherapy

Busulfan. Busulfan has been used for the treatment of CML since 1953. It is always given by mouth, being extremely insoluble. Side effects are minimal in the short run, and there is a high chance that the drug will control the symptoms of CML. Since treatment with busulfan is also inexpensive, it is not surprising that it has become increasingly popular over the years, while older therapeutic alternatives have lost favor. However, busulfan is by no means devoid of danger and must be used cautiously; even then long-term complications of treatment are not uncommon, particularly marrow depression.

Busulfan is an alkylating agent which produces its effect by suppressing the immature myeloid cells. The consequences of this suppression are a gradual disappearance of such cells from the blood, and eventually a fall in the excessive number of mature leukocytes, as well as platelets if these had been increased. Concurrently the hemoglobin level rises. It is emphasized that the changes in the blood count are slow to appear; in fact, with conventional dosages of busulfan, few changes are to be expected in the first 2 weeks, and it is important to resist the temptation to increase the dosage at that stage. Once treatment has been started, the same dosage should be maintained for at least the first 3 weeks. If nothing appears to have happened by then, it is probable that the diagnosis is wrong, and this possibility should be seriously considered before the dose is changed.

Treatment with busulfan should be started in symptomatic patients once the diagnosis of CML has been established. An average daily dose of busulfan is 4 mg given as 2×2 mg tablets, either together or night and morning. This is continued until the leukocyte count has fallen to around $20\,000/\mu l$ and then stopped. The count will continue to fall in most cases and may reach slightly subnormal levels. At the same time the enlarged spleen should regress in size, but this nearly always takes longer than the normalization of the blood count, and several months, as well as several courses of busulfan, may be needed before the spleen becomes impalpable. Diminution of hepatomegaly proceeds concurrently with that of splenomegaly, and the patient's well-being improves and in most cases returns to normal.

Regular blood counts should be made as soon as treatment with busulfan is begun, and continued after the drug has been stopped. Once the count is normal, the period during which it remains so, in the absence of chemotherapy, varies greatly in individual patients, from a few weeks to many months. Eventually the leukocytes and perhaps the platelets rise again, and a second course of busulfan treatment should be started when the count reaches about 30 000/µl. At that stage a daily dose of 2–3 mg may suffice to render the count normal again. Subsequent courses can be given as required, or alternatively a daily maintenance dose sufficient to keep the leukocytes and platelets near their normal levels may be administered. Maintenance doses must be carefully adjusted for each patient to avoid overdosage. They may range from perhaps 2–4 mg per *week* to 4 mg per day, and with such a regimen the disease can be controlled and something like normal health maintained for months to several years, depending on how long the patient remains sensitive to the drug. Gradually, however, it becomes more difficult to maintain normal blood counts and freedom from symptoms, and the dosage of busulfan needs increasing to produce the same effects as could previously be got with a lower one. Eventually a refractory state ensues (see below), when the disease enters the accelerated and much less favorable phase.

The most important *adverse effect* of busulfan is marrow depression. This can happen if too high doses of the drug are given initially, without proper checks on the blood count, or if lower doses are administered for too long. It is most important to realize that, when busulfan is given, once the leukocyte count has started falling, it will continue to do so even after the drug has been stopped, and that there is no way of forecasting the eventual leukocyte and platelet levels in any one patient. For this reason caution is always necessary when busulfan is used. It is better to give too little than too much, because once marrow depression has been induced, leukocyte counts tend to remain abnormally low permanently. Similarly thrombocytopenia and anemia continue indefinitely. Many fatal cases of busulfan myelotoxicity have been described.

Other side effects of long-term busulfan administration also occur and must be looked for early to avoid eventual serious complications. Among the most unfortunate is *pulmonary fibrosis*, a rare but potentially fatal complication. It causes dyspnea, often severe, has characteristic X-ray findings, and may lead to the development of cor pulmonale. Any suspicion that pulmonary fibrosis may be occurring should cause immediate suspension of busulfan therapy.

Pigmentation resembling that of Addison's disease is more common than pulmonary fibrosis. It occurs in as many as one-third of all patients after 2 or more years of busulfan therapy and may be associated with other symptoms suggestive of Addison's disease — debility, lack of appetite, nausea, vomiting, and loss of weight. The pigmentation is brownish and affects the whole body, particularly the trunk, face, and hands. The syndrome differs from Addison's disease in that levels of the various steroid hormones in blood and urine are normal. Early diagnosis is important, so that busulfan can be stopped and severe cachexia avoided.

Other Drugs. Several drugs other than busulfan are available for the treatment of CML, but none have been so widely used. Among the most important are hydroxyurea (HU) and dibromomannitol (DBM). Neither HU nor DBM is obtainable in some countries. They are both given by mouth and appear to have at least one advantage over busulfan, in that both act more quickly and are less likely to cause serious marrow depression due to overdosage. On the other hand relapse of the disease is also quicker to occur after either HU or DBM has been stopped. Not enough is known about either drug to recommend it as

5

being preferable to busulfan, and neither HU nor DBM is likely to be helpful in cases that have become refractory to busulfan.

Radiotherapy

Irradiation of the spleen has been used for the treatment of CML since 1902, that is 50 years longer than chemotherapy. It is an effective means of giving therapy, but since it requires expensive equipment — either ortho- or supravoltage — there are now few centers that have not abandoned it in favor of the much more convenient chemotherapy. The usual way of administering radiotherapy is to give 6–12 treatments of 100 rads each, over a 3- to 4-week period, to the enlarged spleen. This causes few if any adverse symptoms and usually produces rapid shrinkage of the spleen, associated with a fall in leukocyte and platelet counts, a disappearance of immature cells from the blood, and a rise in the hemoglobin level — in short, a remission equivalent in every respect to that produced by chemotherapy. Remissions so caused may last for several to many months, after which further courses of X-ray therapy can be given.

An alternative way of giving radiation therapy is by means of intravenously or orally administered radiophosphorus (P^{32}). In experienced hands this can be very effective, but P^{32} should not be employed by anyone dealing only with occasional cases of CML.

Management of the Refractory Phase

Sooner or later nearly all patients with CML enter a phase that is refractory to all forms of treatment which had hitherto been able to relieve symptoms and maintain the blood count at or near normal levels. The onset of this phase can be recognized either by the fact that treatment is becoming less efficacious and that symptoms such as bleeding — especially petechial rashes — splenomegaly, or anemia are getting worse or by characteristic changes in the blood picture, especially increasing anemia and thrombocytopenia, and the appearance of growing numbers of primitive cells, especially blasts. Clinically and hematologically, this so-called blast crisis closely resembles acute leukemia, but it usually fails to respond to forms of treatment which produce remissions in patients with acute leukemia. If cytogenetic studies are made at this stage, changes resembling those of acute leukemia will generally be found. In addition the Philadelphia chromosome, or sometimes more than one such chromosome, will be seen in most or all dividing cells.

It is now known that there are several varieties of blast crisis which differ from each other in the morphologic and immunologic characteristics of the primitive cells. This is at present of greater theoretical than practical importance, except for the fact that one of the varieties stands out because it is to some degree responsive to relatively simple therapy similar to that given in acute lymphocytic leukemia. It has been found that about one in three patients with blast crisis will obtain a partial or complete remission when prednisone (40–180 mg/day) and vincristine (1–2 mg/m² per week) are given in repeated 2-week courses. Unfortunately such remissions are usually only short, the median duration being about 9 months. Many other forms of chemotherapy, including multidrug combinations, have been tried in blast crisis, but, far from improving the patient's well-being, they have often seemed to hasten death. As a matter of policy, when a patient has been diagnosed as having entered blast crisis it is worthwhile trying the effect of prednisone and vincristine therapy since this combination sometimes produces temporary relief and causes few side effects of its own. However, if this regimen is ineffective, there is little point in proceeding to run the gamut of other chemotherapeutic agents in efforts to obtain a remission. It is better to concentrate on attempts to relieve the patient's symptoms by other means such as analgesics or blood transfusions.

Ancillary Treatment

Besides chemotherapy and radiotherapy a variety of agents are at times helpful in preventing or relieving the symptoms of CML. One of the most common complications in untreated CML is hyperuricemia due to a great increase in the nucleic acid metabolism of the grossly expanded mass of leukocytes. Hyperuricemia may cause the symptoms of gout, renal calculi, and, if prolonged, chronic renal damage. Successful treatment of CML leads to further acceleration of nucleic acid breakdown with a rapid rise in serum and urinary uric acid and consequent danger of acute renal shutdown from tubular blockage by uric acid crystals. It is essential to prevent this catastrophe by increasing the patient's fluid intake and by the administration of allopurinol, which inhibits the formation of uric acid from xanthine and hypoxanthine. A dose of 100–200 mg given orally three times daily is usually sufficient. This should be started as soon as the diagnosis of CML is clear and before chemotherapy is given. Once the cell mass has been reduced, allopurinol can also be reduced and ultimately discontinued.

Blood transfusions are usually not required until the later stages since successful chemotherapy relieves the anemia which is commonly found in patients with CML. Some patients, however, present with severe anemia, and small transfusions may give them an initial boost. Large single transfusions should never be given as they may cause a sudden rise in blood viscosity which may already be higher than normal because of a greatly increased leukocyte concentration. In blast crisis transfusion can be one of the few ways of relieving the patient's feelings of weakness, tiredness, and shortness of breath. It is a matter of fine judgment how long one should continue transfusing a patient who is failing rapidly.

Prognosis

The prognosis of CML is uniformly bad: although survival times vary, death is the inevitable outcome. In this respect, there has been no change in the prognosis since treatment capable of producing remissions first became generally available at the beginning of the century. This dismal situation contrasts with that in acute leukemia, whose prognosis has improved startlingly: whereas it was hopeless until the late 1940s, the outlook is now one of probable cure for many children and some adults. It is thus fair to say that, of all types of leukemia, CML has presently the worst prognosis for survival. No radical improvement in the prognosis is in view.

As has been seen above, however, treatment is capable of relieving the symptoms of CML in most patients and thereby of adding greatly to the quality of their remaining lives. Treatment can also cause a modest prolongation of life in some patients. The result of treatment, properly given, is then that the patient can return to his usual occupation and way of living and can carry on with it for months or years. In large series of CML patients published in recent years the median survival time has varied between 3 and 4 years. This is some 6–18 months longer than the prognosis usually quoted before the introduction of chemotherapy. The factor limiting the effectiveness of treatment in most cases is the onset of blast crisis which is resistant to most forms of chemotherapy and to radiotherapy. Indeed the variability of survival times is almost entirely due to variations in the interval between the original diagnosis of CML and the onset of blast crisis. For reasons which are not understood, this interval is prolonged in occasional patients who may therefore live for 10 or more years in reasonable health. It seems likely that such long survivals are determined more by the inherent nature of the disease in these patients than by the type of treatment employed.

Chronic Lymphocytic Leukemia

Clinical Picture

In contrast to CML, CLL gives rise to few symptoms in the earlier stages and can remain entirely asymptomatic for many years. For this reason CLL is often discovered accidentally, when a blood count is done for some unconnected purpose. At that stage there may be few or no abnormal physical signs, and the question then arises whether what seems to be an abnormal blood count indicates the presence of leukemia. This used to be a question which only the efflux of time — sometimes considerable periods — could settle. Recent progress in the immunology of leukemias and lymphomas has made it easier to determine whether mild changes in the blood count are the early signs of CLL.

In some patients CLL is not only clinically silent when it is first discovered but it also progresses very slowly. Indeed the course of the disease can be so prolonged that death may occur from an intercurrent cause, rather than from the leukemia. CLL is largely a disease of old people who are at increased risk of dying from many other causes. One such is cancer. As CLL occurs in the "cancer age" some patients may be expected to develop a second malignancy during the course of their leukemia. There are in fact good statistics to show that patients with CLL are more prone to have cancer than their nonleukemic contemporaries. Symptoms which arise in patients with CLL may therefore be due to another cancer rather than the leukemia and may cause difficult diagnostic problems.

Once abnormal physical signs arise in CLL, the most common are the following:

1. Lymphadenopathy. This is usually widespread, particularly in the cervical, axillary, and inguinal areas. The nodes are mildly to moderately enlarged, soft, discrete, and painless. Investigation may show that deep-seated groups such as those in the mediastinum and abdomen are also enlarged, usually moderately.
2. Splenomegaly. This often accompanies lymphadenopathy. The spleen is usually mildly to moderately enlarged and firm but not hard; however, in occasional cases it is disproportionately large and may appear to fill the abdomen. In such cases there can be discomfort, but usually splenic infarction does not occur. Hepatomegaly may occur at the same time as splenomegaly.
3. General symptoms such as fever, fatigue, and weight loss appear in the late stages.

Patients with advanced CLL have an increased susceptibility to infections, especially respiratory, and this may cause considerable distress toward the end. Herpes zoster is another frequent and unpleasant complication. Autoimmune hemolytic anemia occurs in some 10% and autoimmune thrombocytopenic purpura less frequently. Skin lesions of many varieties are more common in CLL than in other types of leukemia.

Laboratory Investigations

The most characteristic abnormality is a *lymphocytosis* which may range from 15 to 600×10^9/liter or even higher. The lymphocytes are small and mature in the great majority of cases, and morphologically indistinguishable from normal lymphocytes. Immunologically these cells are B-lymphocytes in more than 95% of patients, and where immunoglobulin allotypes can be determined, it is found that the cells all carry a single heavy and a single light chain; this signifies that the lymphocytes are derived from a common precursor and, in fact, they form a single clone, like other malignant cells. The finding of such a clone confirms the diagnosis of CLL (cf. above). In a small proportion of cases (less than 5%) the lymphocytes are a clone of T cells, not B cells. Such cases have an atypical clinical course and are resistant to therapy.

Anemia is absent or mild in the earlier stages of CLL. When it develops later, it is normocytic and normochromic and becomes progressively more severe. In about 10% of patients signs of hemolysis such as spherocytosis, reticulocytosis, a positive direct antiglobulin (Coombs) test, bilirubinemia, and a low serum haptoglobin are found.

Hypogammaglobulinemia occurs in most patients with CLL, often from the early stages. IgG, IgM, and IgA may all be diminished, but sometimes there is a diffuse increase in IgG, occasionally associated with a monoclonal paraprotein peak. The *bone marrow* is generally infiltrated with the same small lymphocytes as those in the blood, at first focally but later in a diffuse manner. In the late stages the marrow becomes "packed" with lymphocytes, and there develops suppression of the normal blood cell precursors, with ensuing pancytopenia.

As stated above, the early stages of CLL may be difficult to diagnose with certainty, but as the disease progresses its character becomes more obvious, and in the later stages there is scarcely any need, in most cases, for tests other than blood counts, to establish the diagnosis.

Whereas an acute transformation (blast crisis) is the common terminal even in CML, a similar transformation in CLL is practically unknown. However, there may be the development of a second malignancy of the blood, namely *acute* leukemia. This can be a consequence of the increased susceptibility of CLL patients to cancer or, alternatively, it may be induced by the chemotherapy or radiotherapy that has been given. In either case, the onset of acute leukemia is likely to be a late and rapidly fatal event.

Management

Principles

The most important problem in the management of CLL is not *how* to treat the condition, but *whether* or *when* to treat it. This at first sight paradoxical problem arises from two facts:

1. Many patients have no symptoms or only few symptoms when CLL is diagnosed and for long afterward.
2. It is not known whether treatment of asymptomatic patients or those with only minor manifestations of CLL confers any benefit on them. Where there are no symptoms, they do not need relieving. If early treatment were able to postpone the onset of symptoms or to prolong life in the long run, its administration might be justified. However, the evidence on these points is so far equivocal.

The great American hematologist William Dameshek suggested nearly 20 years ago that CLL was an "accumulative disease," by which he meant that its manifestations were due to a gradual piling up of lymphocytes in organs where they eventually interfered with normal functioning. Among such organs was the marrow, which would become incapable of producing normal blood cells, but any other organ could be similarly affected. Dameshek also proposed that the accumulating lymphocytes were abnormal and incapable of fulfilling their normal immunologic function such as defense against infection. The main implication of these suggestions was the prediction that the natural history of CLL would be one of steady and inevitable deterioration, and this has been amply borne out by subsequent studies.

It is now clear that cases of CLL can be classified according to the *stage* the disease has reached at diagnosis and that it is that stage which largely determines the further outlook for each patient. Table 3 shows the first of several staging systems for CLL (the "Rai" system).

Table 3 indicates the gradual progression of CLL from a very chronic disease (stage 0) to one that is rapidly fatal (stages III and IV). For example, a patient diagnosed purely on the strength of a lymphocytosis (stage 0) can generally expect to live for many years; if the diagnosis is not made until there is anemia as well as hepatosplenomegaly (stage III), the median life expectancy is less than 2 years. It should be noted that all the figures are medians, and that there are considerable differences in the speed with which individual patients pass through the series of stages and in the length of time they spend in each stage. These differences depend on the aggressiveness of the disease process or its indolence in each patient.

The most generally accepted therapeutic principle in CLL is to give treatment for the relief of symptoms only. The more aggressive the disease process, the more likely is it that

Table 3. Clinical staging system for CLL

Stage	Main features at diagnosis	Outlook (median survival time in months)
0	Lymphocytosis in blood ($>15 \times 10^9$/liter) and marrow ($>40\%$)	Over 150
I	Stage 0 plus lymphadenopathy	101
II	Stage 0 plus splenomegaly, hepatomegaly, or both	71
III	Stage 0 plus anemia (Hb<110 g/liter)	19
IV	Stage 0 plus thrombocytopenia (platelets $<100 \times 10^9$/liter)	19
0–IV		71

Table 4. Symptoms indicating need for treatment in CLL

1.	Evidence of bone marrow failure — anemia, neutropenia, thrombocytopenia
2.	Development of autoimmune hemolytic anemia or autoimmune thrombocytopenic purpura
3.	Presence of splenomegaly that is causing symptoms, or evidence of hypersplenism
4.	Presence of symptoms due to lymphadenopathy, or involvement of skin or solid organs
5.	Repeated infections

the patient will develop symptoms sooner rather than later, and hence that treatment will be required. Lymphadenopathy of more than minimal degree will, for instance, usually be an indication for treatment, as will the onset of significant anemia. Whether, however, patients with mild lymphadenopathy and splenomegaly but no anemia should be treated in the absence of definite symptoms is another matter. It could be argued that treatment in such cases might reduce the stage of the patient's disease from II to I or from I to 0 and so improve the long-term outlook, but it is not clear at present if such changes imply concomitant changes (for the better) in the prognosis. In the absence of such information most clinicians currently restrict their therapy in CLL to the management of symptomatic patients. Table 4 gives a list of the principal symptom complexes which indicate the need for treatment.

When a patient with CLL is seen for the first time, the doctor should ask himself a number of questions before deciding on the treatment to be employed:

1. Are symptoms present?
2. Are they severe enough to demand urgent relief?
3. How long have they been present?
4. Can the rate of progress of the disease be estimated?

If no symptoms are present, no treatment need be given for the time being, but the patient should be kept under regular observation, with blood counts every 3–6 months. If severe symptoms are present, treatment should be begun without delay; its nature is discussed below. In the intermediate group, treatment can usually be postponed until it is clearer how rapidly the disease is progressing. This may mean a delay of from several weeks to several months, at the end of which the aim should be to give the minimal treatment likely to relieve symptoms and, if possible, to inhibit the progress of the disease which has been observed. Minimization of treatment is indicated because most CLL patients are elderly and therefore not only prone to complicating disease, but also less able to tolerate the side effects of therapy, which can be more significant than those of the leukemia.

Chemotherapy

Chemotherapy for CLL became feasible in the 1950s, at about the same time as that for CML. In contrast to CML, there are two chief groups of agents, alkylating agents and adrenal corticosteroid hormones, both active against this type of leukemia. They produce their effects by different mechanisms and are therefore often used in combination.

Alkylating Agents. Chronic lymphocytic leukemia will respond in some degree to almost any alkylating agent, including busulfan, but that chosen most frequently is *chlorambucil*

11

(Leukeran) because it has a selective action on cells of the lymphoid compared with the myeloid series, is easily given by mouth, has few side effects, at least in the short run, and is also inexpensive. Chlorambucil is given as tablets in daily doses of 0.1–0.2 mg/kg body weight, preferably before breakfast to improve absorption. The course is continued until a maximal effect is obtained and is then stopped. Effects to be expected in the majority of patients are a gradual improvement in well-being, with subsidence of fever and gains in appetite and weight. Simultaneously there is a fall in the leukocytosis and diminution in lymphadenopathy, and, less constantly, in hepatosplenomegaly. The effects on the white cells fall largely, though not entirely, on the lymphocytes, which gradually return to somewhere near normal figures. However, it is uncommon for the blood count to become completely normal, and some degree of lymphocytosis persists in many cases. In the marrow the lymphocytosis also diminishes in many instances, but a complete remission, with normalization of the marrow, is extremely rare. Anemia and thrombocytopenia, if present, often do not improve with chlorambucil treatment, and neither does hypogammaglobulinemia.

Once the lymphocyte count has returned to a near-normal level, chlorambucil is best discontinued until a significant further rise in lymphocytes has occurred. This may happen within a few months, after which treatment can be begun again. The choice now lies between a second course of chlorambucil at the same or a slightly reduced dose rate or an attempt to put the patient on a small maintenance dose (1–4 mg/day). If a limited course of the drug is given, this is discontinued when the count has fallen to a near-normal level, with subsequent similar courses. Maintenance therapy is given continuously, with the aim of achieving a gradual return of the count to normal and keeping it there. Regular blood counts must be done whichever method is chosen, in order to prevent the untoward effects of overdosage.

The most important *adverse effect* of chlorambucil is marrow depression, with consequent neutropenia, anemia, and thrombocytopenia. Since many patients in the later stages of CLL have depressed marrows in any case as the result of their disease, the addition of chlorambucil is apt to aggravate this condition; as a result less of the drug can be given than would be desirable for the treatment of the lymphocyte infiltration. Combined treatment with adrenal corticosteroids can often prevent this harmful effect of chlorambucil given alone (see below). There are few other adverse effects of chlorambucil administration.

A number of physicians prefer *cyclophosphamide* to chlorambucil in the therapy for CLL because it is less likely to cause thrombocytopenia. It can be given in short courses of large intravenous doses but is more often used as oral maintenance doses of 50–150 mg/day. Unlike chlorambucil, cyclophosphamide may cause nausea, vomiting, and alopecia, but its most characteristic toxic effect is hemorrhagic cystitis, a very distressing symptom. As mentioned above, almost all other alkylating agents have some effect in CLL, but none are as predictable or so relatively free from side effects as chlorambucil. For this reason they are not at present recommended.

Adrenal Corticosteroid Hormones. These have long been known to be capable of causing destruction of lymphoid tissue, both normal and leukemic. They do so not, like the alkylating agents, by interfering with the division of immature cell precursors, but by a direct action on mature lymphocytes and on no other blood or marrow cells. Because of this mechanism, they are the only class of agents that does not cause marow depression.

When marrow depression is present as a result of infiltration by leukemic lymphocytes, this can be diminished by the giving of steroids, so that the myeloid and erythroid precursors and megakaryocytes can once again fulfil their normal function of replenishing stocks of mature cells. Hence steroid administration not only destroys leukemic cells but relieves anemia, neutropenia, and thrombocytopenia.

Adrenal corticosteroid hormones may be used whenever therapy for CLL is required but are especially valuable in the later stages. It is often a good plan to begin treatment with prednisone or prednisolone (the most commonly used and least expensive of the steroids) in oral doses such as 0.5–1.0 mg/kg/day and to add chlorambucil in about 2 weeks. In many cases the steroids produce an extremely rapid and almost visible shrinkage of the enlarged lymphoid organs, both nodes and spleen. At the same time, the lymphocyte count tends to *rise* temporarily, because of a redistribution of the lymphocytes in the body. A high lymphocytosis can persist for several weeks but is followed by a fall toward normal, especially once chlorambucil has been added. At the same time, the marrow shows a lessening infiltration with lymphocytes. Because of the rapid destruction of large masses of lymphoid tissues there is a particular danger of hyperuricemia and its consequences when steroids are given, and allopurinol should always be used together with them (see above).

Although adrenal corticosteroid hormones have the great advantage of causing no marrow depression, they have many other well-known toxic effects which are of particular importance at the advanced ages at which CLL occurs. Among these are fluid retention, cardiac failure, diabetes mellitus, osteoporosis, peptic ulceration, and psychiatric disturbances. Where any of these are present before treatment steroids should be given with great caution, and in any case total doses should be carefully limited. There is no possibility of indefinite steroid administration, and the usual practice is to give short courses of a few weeks at a time. Twice weekly of alternate daily doses of 1–2 mg/kg are said to be less dangerous than smaller daily ones. A careful watch must be kept for the reactivation of any preexisting tuberculous lesions, and appropriate antibiotics prescribed in case this should occur.

Steroids are of particular value in cases where autoimmune hemolytic anemia or thrombocytopenia develops. These conditions usually require high doses of prednisone which may need to be given intermittently for long periods. Immunosuppressive drugs such as azathioprine or 6-mercaptopurine are occasionally useful in supplementing steroids. Splenectomy may be indicated when hemolysis persists in spite of long-term intermittent steroid therapy (see below).

Radiotherapy

Radiotherapy has been used in the treatment of CLL as long as in that of CML. The usual form is irradiation of either enlarged lymph nodes or the spleen. Small doses are highly effective in causing rapid involution of these organs, but the general effects of such treatment — particularly on the blood count — are less uniform or predictable. Localized irradiation is still used today to provide fast relief where large lymphoid masses cause distressing symptoms or are cosmetically objectionable, but as an alternative to chemotherapy it has few attractions. However, total body irradiation has lately been tried and appears to have a definite place, especially when patients with CLL have become resistant to chemotherapy. Total body irradiation is a simple and often effective form of

Table 5. Indications for splenectomy in CLL

1.	Autoimmune hemolytic anemia unresponsive to steroids or immunodepressive drugs or needing treatment with excessively high doses of steroids
2.	Autoimmune thrombocytopenia in similar circumstances
3.	Evidence of hypersplenism
4.	Gross splenomegaly giving rise to severe symptoms and unresponsive to drugs

radiotherapy which can be given with orthovoltage equipment. The patient sits or stands in the beam, the uniformity of the field depending on the distance at which irradiation is applied. Four doses of 10–15 rads each are often sufficient to produce marked improvement in symptoms and in the blood count, and such short courses can be repeated as necessary, a maximum total dose being 150–300 rads. Side effects are absent or minimal. Total body irradiation, where it is available, probably deserves a place in the treatment of symptomatic advanced CLL resistant to chemotherapy.

Ancillary Treatment

Blood transfusions are frequently required for patients with CLL and marrow depression and especially when there is autoimmune hemolytic anemia. Marrow-depressed patients present a chronic problem that calls for the regular administration of small to moderate (2–4 units) quantities of blood or packed red cells. Hemolysis can be sudden and devastating and can give rise to acute transfusion problems of great severity, especially when there are difficulties in obtaining compatible blood. High-dose steroids are often necessary as an aid in overcoming these difficulties.

The treatment of hypogammaglobulinemia may cause one of the most prominent and persistent therapeutic dilemmas in advanced CLL. The almost constant infections which such patients suffer can be most wearing for them. Antibiotics are almost continuously required but often fail to clear up recurrent respiratory and other infections. The prophylactic administration of pooled human gamma globulin at 2–4 weekly intervals, especially in the winter months, has often been tried, and some patients have reported diminutions in the frequency of their infections. However, such preparations have to be given intramuscularly, which restricts the size of the injections, and there is also a risk of serum hepatitis and allergic reactions. Intravenous preparations of human gamma globulin are not generally available and are very expensive.

Splenectomy has an occasional place in the treatment of CLL, but its use should be restricted to situations where there is a clear indication, as shown in Table 5.

The diagnosis of hypersplenism theoretically requires demonstration that the spleen abnormally sequesters red cells or platelets, but this is not always possible. In such circumstances splenectomy may be justified for the treatment of refractory nonhemolytic anemia or thrombocytopenia provided the patient is fit enough to undergo a major operation.

Prognosis

Chronic lymphocytic leukemia has long had the reputation of being a relatively innocuous form of leukemia which may cause little trouble for many of those who have it. This is true to the extent that elderly people diagnosed in stages O or I may well die from other causes before CLL has advanced to the point where it causes significant symptoms. On the other hand the statistical investigations of recent years have made it clear that, given enough time for the accumulation of the leukemic cells, most if not all CLLs have the capacity for causing symptoms and eventual death. Thus CLL will amost certainly shorten the survival of patients discovered to have it in their forties or fifties. Moreover, the symptoms of advanced CLL nearly always cause considerable distress, so that death may finally come as a relief. An overall median survival of 4–6 years from diagnosis is evidence that, for many, CLL is a grave disease. As has been seen, treatment of CLL is still basically unsatisfactory. Although symptoms may be relieved and the quality of life improved, there is still room for doubt whether or how much presently available therapeutic modalities extend life. Research to provide new ways of treating CLL is, more than ever, of the utmost importance.

Further Reading

Canellos GP (1982) Chronic leukemias. In: DeVita VT, Hellman S, Rosenberg SA (eds) Cancer: Principles of practice of oncology. Lippincott, Philadelphia, pp 1427–1438

Galton DAG, Szur WL, Dacie JV (1961) The use of chlorambucil and steroids in the treatment of chronic lymphocytic leukemia. Br J Haematol 7: 73–98

Karanas A, Silver RT (1968) Characteristics of the terminal phase of chronic granulocytic leukemia. Blood 32: 445

Spiers ASD (1975) New approaches to the therapy of chronic granulocytic leukemia. Series Haematol 8: 157

2. Acute Leukemia in Adults

E. S. Henderson

Introduction

Acute leukemia in adults comes in many varieties which can be distinguished by differences in leukemic cell morphology, immunologic characteristics, cytogenetics, response to treatment, and complications. All forms, however, are characterized by progressive infiltration of blood-forming organs — in particular of the bone marrow — which leads to pancytopenia and infection, bleeding, weakness, and fatigue. The management of all forms requires that marrow function be restored to normal. At present this must be achieved by maximum reduction of leukemia cells throughout the body by combinations of antileukemic drugs. However, cytotoxic regimens vary in their ability to achieve cytoreduction of the different subtypes; thus diagnosis and subclassification are of primary importance to successful treatment and must be achieved as quickly as possible, *before* embarking upon the definitive treatment program.

Diagnosis

Acute leukemia must be suspected in any patient with sustained and/or progressive abnormalities in the production of any or all blood cells. Its onset may be sudden and explosive or subtle and insidious. Weakness, weight loss, recurrent or unremiting infection, increased bruising, and bleeding from the gums or petechiae are the most common complaints. Less commonly enlarged lymph nodes, subcutaneous nodes, liver, or spleen may be the initial manifestations. Anemia, granulocytopenia, and thrombocytopenia almost always occur but may initially be isolated abnormalities. Eventually, however, all normal blood cells are reduced. It must be stressed that leukemia occurs often *without elevation* of blood counts, and on rare occasions without clearly abnormal leukocytes being identified in the peripheral blood smears. Because of this a bone marrow examination is essential for proper diagnosis.

When the diagnosis of leukemia is established or strongly suspected, the specific subtype must be clarified. In order to do so, whenever possible a bone marrow aspirate and biopsy should be obtained. The first few drops of the aspirate should be used to make six or more marrow smears for morphologic and cytochemical assessment. An additional milliliter should be injected into media for cellular and cytogenetic study, and a final milliliter is fixed in Zenker's solution, centrifuged, and the pellet sectioned for histologic evaluation. If the facilities for immunologic characterization are available, marrow or blood leukemic cells should be collected (by marrow aspiration and venipuncture respectively), suspended in medium containing preservative-free heparin, and assayed for surface and cytoplasm immunoglobulins, sheep erythrocyte receptors, the common acute lymphoblastic leukemia antigen (CALLA), and, if monoclonal antibodies are available, for Ia-like, T cell, and myeloid antigens.

Morphologic and cytochemical criteria should be used to determine the illness's place in the French-American-British (FAB) classification scheme (see Tables 1, 2). For this, the essential stains are a Romanovsky (Wright's, or Wright-Giemsa) stain, periodic acid — Schiff (PAS) peroxidase, nonspecific esterase, and acid phosphatase. In about three-fourths of cases distinction of subclasses can be made on the basis or morphology alone. In the remainder, and especially for undifferentiated leukemias and the L_1 and M_1 FAB categories, cytochemistry is helpful, but immunologic and cytogenetic studies are often required. Major variations in treatment exist between acute lymphoblastic leukemia (ALL) of the "common," non-T and non-B variety, other forms of ALL (T cell and B cell), and acute myeloid leukemia. These entities can be differentiated morphologically and histochemically in most cases. B-cell ALL can be identified more conclusively by the

Table 1. Scoring system for acute lymphoblastic leukemia

Criteria	Score
High N/C ratio $\geqslant 75\%$ of cells	+
Low N/C ratio $\geqslant 25\%$ of cells	—
Nucleoli: 0 to 1 (small) $\geqslant 75\%$ of cells	+
Nucleoli: 1 or more prominent $\geqslant 25\%$ of cells	—
Irregular nuclear membrane $\geqslant 25\%$ of cells	—
Large cells $\geqslant 50\%$ of cells	—

L_1 = total score of 0 to 2+
L_2 = total score of —1 to —4

N/C, × nuclear cytoplasmic ratio
L_3, large uniform basophilic cells with round nuclei, dense granular chromatin, and one or more prominent nucleoli

Table 2. Criteria for acute myeloid leukemia subtypes

Bone marrow cells	M_1	M_2	M_4	M_5	M_6
Blasts	%	%	%	%	%
All nucleated cells	–	> 30	> 30	–	< 30 or > 30
Nonerythroid cells	90 (I+II)	> 30	> 30	> 80	> 30
Erythroblasts, all nucleated cells	–	< 50	> 50	–	> 50
Granulocytic component	< 10	> 10	> 20	< 20	Variable
Monocytic component	< 10	< 20	> 20	> 80	Variable

M_3, hypergranular promyelocytic leukemia

18

presence of monoclonal immunoglobulin on the cell surface, while cell disease can be distinguished by the binding of unsensitized sheep red blood cells to form "E rosettes," or more precisely through the use of monoclonal antibodies.

Preliminary Therapy

While a precise diagnosis is being established it is important to prepare the patient for the rigorous type-specific antileukemia therapy which will shortly follow. This preparation centers upon three areas of pathology:

1. Defects in blood cell formation
2. Products of leukemic cells
3. Concomitant organ system dysfunctions, related or unrelated to the leukemia, which will complicate treatment

Correction of these abnormalities is, at this stage, necessarily partial and temporary, complete correction depending on full control of disease manifestations, i. e., induction of complete remission.

Defects of Blood Cell Production

Severe anemia, i. e., a hemoglobin level of less than 9.0 g/100 ml should always be corrected to preserve optimal function of vital organs, particularly the brain, heart, liver, and kidneys. Packed red cell transfusions are generally preferred, since in most cases other blood components and intravenous infusions of medications and fluids will be required and the total volume of infusion becomes an important consideration. It is not necessary to reestablish normal levels of hemoglobin or hematocrit — a range of 9–11 is usually safe and readily accomplished.

Platelet transfusions sufficient to maintain blood platelet concentrations above $20\,000/\mu l$ will usually forestall dangerous hemorrhage. In most patients who are afebrile and have not built up platelet antibodies this can be achieved by administration of platelets obtained from 4 units of blood, repeated every 2–3 days or more frequently as needed. Again, it is preferable for donor and recipient alike to use platelet concentrates, unless there is a specific need for fresh plasma, as in patients with disseminated intravascular coagulation. The risk of hemorrhage is increased in patients who are febrile, for whom transfusions should be given more frequently and at higher platelet doses.

Transfusions of normal granulocytes are valuable in patients who have sustained granylocytopenia together with sepsis or other systemic infection unreponsive to broad spectrum antibiotics. This is usually not the case at the time of diagnosis.

Leukemic Cell Hyperproliferation

Excessive numbers of immature leukemic cells can cause severe disease by two mechanisms in addition to inhibition of production of normal blood cells. First of all, leukemic cells can migrate from the blood and marrow into all organs of the body. These infiltrates,

19

surprisingly, are frequently asymptomatic, and rarely require special treatment. However, infiltrates can impair venous blood flow, e. g., in the superior vena cava, or fluid outflow from the spinal fluid space in patients with meningeal leukemia. These are seldom presenting problems, but in the rare circumstances when symptomatic infiltrate does occur they can be treated with low dose local radiation treatment, followed, in the case of meningeal leukemia, by intrathecal medication before or concomitant with specific therapy. This will be dealt with in the section on remission maintenance.

A more serious emergency exists when the blast cell count in the blood is high and rapidly rising. In such a circumstance, commonest with T cell ALL and with monoblastic (M_5) or myelomonocytic (M_4) forms of AML, small arteries and arterioles become plugged with masses of blast cells. This is associated with invasion of vessel walls, local anoxia, and hemorrhage. These leukostatic lesions are rare with blood blast cell counts less than 150 000/µl, and are of major consequence only in the lungs and the brain. Leukostasis in these organs, however, can have devastating and frequently lethal sequelae: acute respiratory distress syndrome and massive intracerebral hemorrhage. The threat of leukostasis is reduced as the blast cell count is lowered. This can be accomplished in virtually all cases by the intravenous administration of hydroxyurea 3 g/m^2 repeated in 12–24 h if the blast cell count has not fallen below 100 000/µl. Alternatively, cyclophosphamide 1 g/m^2 by i. v. bolus or cytosine arabinoside 200–500 mg/m^2 by continuous infusion for 1–4 h is similarly effective. If a continuous flow cell separator is available, the blast cell count can be reduced by frequent leukapheresis. This method has the advantage of removing a large mass of leukemia cells before they can release their intracellular urates, phosphates, sulfates, and procoagulants into the patient's bloodstream (see below). Cytotoxic drugs, on the other hand, do not require special blood collection equipment, do not usually require concomitant anticoagulation, and do not immediately reduce platelet levels to the extent observed with multiple leuka pheresis. Either method of rapid reduction of the blast cell count is temporary and accordingly specific treatment of the leukemia must be started as soon as possible after the emergency measures have been instituted.

Products of Leukemic Cells

Uric Acid

Cell death and nucleic acid turnover are accelerated in all forms of acute leukemia. As a consequence, uric acid production and uric acid pools increase dramatically. Uric acid is excreted in the urine, and concentrations in the urine can easily exceed saturation limits, leading to precipitation of urates in renal tubules and renal failure. The risk of this complication is increased with dehydration and acidosis, and temporarily with effective cytolytic chemotherapy.

Prevention of uric acid nephropathy is simple and effective if undertaken early. Immediately upon diagnosis, abundant fluids should be provided orally and, if necessary, intravenously, so as to ensure an hourly urine flow of 100 ml/h throughout the full day (24 hours). Whenever hydration is uncertain, fluids should be adminstered by continuous round-the-clock intravenous infusions until the uric acid levels are lowered and the bulk of leukemia has been markedly reduced. Allopurinol (5-hydroxypyrazolopyrimidine) should be started simultaneously with hydration. A dose of 100 mg/m^2 every 8 h is usually sufficient, but if the serum uric acid concentration does not fall within 48 h, the dose should be increased to 200 mg/m^2 every 8 h. Some 5% of patients develop allergic reactions to allopurinol. If these are not overly severe, allopurinol should be continued. Otherwişe, urine output should be maintained by intravenous infusions and alkalinization with about 44 mEq/liter of sodium bicarbonate given every 8 h, i. e., one ampule per liter of i. v. fluids. In patients with adequate or increased hydration, adequate serum sodium concentrations, but persistently acid urine, acetazolamide 500 mg orally will increase the urine pH. This effect will be lost as sodium is depleted, but when combined with sodium bicarbonate administration it can tide patients over the critical period — the critical period being the first days of treatment in patients who (a) present with signs of incipient uric acid nephropathy (high serum and urine urate levels, acid urine, and reduced urine flow despite adequate hydration), or (b) prove to be allergic to allopurinol. Full blown uric acid nephropathy can occasionally be prevented in oliguric patients by the infusion of mannitol over 1 h, together with continuation of the above-described measures. Fully established nephropathy will require a renal failure program, including renal dialysis, and tailoring of antileukemia therapy to exclude drugs (methotrexate, 6-mercaptopurine, cyclophosphamide) whose detoxification or elimination depends on renal excretion.

Hypercalcemia

Hypercalcemia is an infrequent complication of acute leukemia in relapse. When present it is generally a result of leukemic cell osteoclast activating factor production, which can be rapidly diminished by cytolytic agents, particularly prednisone. Calcitonin infusions can also be helpful. The condition reverses as remission is approached.

Procoagulants

Leukemic progranulocytes and, to a lesser extent, myeloblasts contain large amounts of procoagulants. Release of these substances in large amounts can overwhelm the normal hemostatic mechanisms of the body, resulting in intravascular consumption and deletion of fibrinogen, factor VIII, factor V, and platelets. Unless corrected this disseminated intravascular coagulation (DIC) can result in devastating hemorrhage throughout the body. Like uric acid nephropathy, DIC is aggravated initially by successful cytolytic therapy, although achieving a remission is the only successful therapy in the long run. As part of the initial pretreatment workup, the partial thromboplastin time, prothrombin time, plasma fibrinogen, and fibrin degradation products (FDPs) should be assayed. Patients with any form of acute leukemia who have low or falling fibrinogen and elevated FDPs should receive heparin 5000 units i. v. every 6 h plus fresh plasma to provide safe levels of labile clotting factors. It must be recognized that fibrinogen levels in the absence of DIC are elevated in acute leukemia. Thus a low normal fibrinogen level associated with elevated FDP levels strongly suggests DIC. Any patient with acute progranulocytic leukemia (APL) (M$_3$ according to the FAB classification) should receive low dose heparin automatically (together with fresh plasma as needed) because of the very high likelihood of DIC during the remission induction period. A non-M$_3$ form of APL with small primary granules but a similar predisposition to DIC can be identified cytogenetically: both standard APL and "microgranular" APL frequently have a specific translocation, t (15 : 17).

If this translocation is identified, patients should receive low dose heparin. However, results of cytogenetic analysis will rarely be available before treatment; therefore, patients with acute nonlymphoblastic leukemia other than M_3-APL should be watched closely for falling fibrinogen levels and rising FDP levels and, if these are noted, treatment with low dose heparin and clotting factor replacement should be commenced.

Other Products

Leukemic cells, like all others, have high concentrations of magnesium, calcium, potassium, phosphates, and sulfates which, when suddenly released into the blood plasma through cytolysis, may cause severe electrolyte intolerance. This can occur early in the successful treatment of all types of leukemia but is most common in ALL when susceptible lymphoblasts are rapidly lysed by corticosteroids. This can precipitate acidosis and cardiac arrythmias, including cardiac arrest.

Concomitant Medical Problems

Remission induction therapy is always stressful and of uncertain outcome. In order to increase the chance of successful outcome the function of all organ systems must be checked and as many deficiencies corrected as is possible. Diabetes mellitus, heart failure, hypo- and hyperthyroidism, and the like should be brought under at least reasonable control and carefully monitored through antileukemia treatment. Fluid overload and hyperglycemia are difficult problems given the need for hydration, the presence of malignant disease, and the use of drugs such as prednisone, vincristine, and asparaginase which induce hyperglycemia and sodium and water retention. The success of treatment often depends as much upon the therapist's skill in general medical management as upon the specific drug regimen used to eliminate leukemic cells.

Any infection should be diagnosed and treatment started before or simultaneous with the start of remission induction therapy. It should be kept in mind that fever is a very rare sign of acute leukemia but is a very common finding in infection.

Occasionally, fever may be seen with dehydration and within 5–6 h following a blood cell transfusion. However, unless clearly associated with one of the above, and unless infection is doubtful clinically on other grounds, a temperature elevation to 38.5° (or above) should be assumed to be of bacterial origin, and broad spectrum antibodies should be started (see p. 28).

It is my practice before and during remission induction to give prophylactic oral antibiotics to reduce the gastrointestinal flora. My preference is trimethoprim-sulfamethoxazole, two tablets t. i. d. until the peripheral blood granulocyte (PMN) count is more than 1000/µl.

The goal of remission induction regimens is to restore rapidly normal marrow function by eliminating leukemic cells. This can be done relatively more easily in non-B, non-T lymphoblastic disease than with myeloblastic disease, as it requires less severely myelosuppressive drugs. The induction regimens for ALL and AML as a consequence differ significantly.

Acute Lymphoblastic Leukemia

Remission Induction

Induction treatment for ALL (and acute undifferentiated leukemia) is based on the additive effects of corticosteroids and vincristine. For poor prognosis categories best results are obtained when asparaginase and an anthracycline are added. Treatment in all forms of ALL in adults should include these four categories of drugs. The regimen I recommend is as follows: *vincristine* 2 mg i. v. weekly ×4 doses, *prednisone* 40 mg/m^2 twice daily for 4 weeks, *daunorubicin* 30 g/m^2 i. v. on each of the first 3 days of the induction period, and *asparaginase* 5000 units/m^2 i. v. daily for the 10 days immediately following the fourth (and last) dose of vincristine.

These drugs need not and should not be reduced because of low blood counts, as bone marrow cytoreduction is necessary early on, and, after the three daunorubicin doses, the remainder of the regimen is only mildly myelosuppressive. Drug doses may need to be reduced in various conditions, dealt with individually below..

Liver Dysfunction

Dosage of vincristine and of daunorubicin should be reduced by half (1 mg and 15 mg/m^2 respectively) for moderate liver excretory function deficits as evidenced by a serum bilirubin level of 1.5–4.0 mg/100 ml.If bilirubin rises to above that level then these drugs, as well as asparaginase, should be withheld in order to avoid severe bone marrow, central nervous system, and cardiac toxicity.

Cardiac Disease

Patients with diffuse myocardial injury and/or weakness, i. e., ventricular ejection fractions of below 40%, clinical congestive heart failure, or recent myocardial infarction should not receive the anthracycline.

Peptic Ulcer Disease or Steroid-Induced Psychosis

A well documented history or the appearance of these complications should contraindicate the use of steroids.

Coagulopathy, Pancreatitis

Asparaginase can cause or aggravate both of these conditions. It should be withheld pending the resolution of pancreatitis, and should be stopped if fibrinogenopenic bleeding unresponsive to clotting factor replacement develops. Fibrinogenopenia alone occurs in almost all patients receiving asparaginase, but as it is usually entirely reversible, asymptomatic, and harmless, asparaginase administration need not be withheld or reduced in most cases.

Other toxicities or the presence of infections, impaired renal or pulmonary function, obtundation, hypercalcemia, hypernatremia, hyperglycemia, bleeding, and so forth, require prompt measures of diagnosis, support, and correction, but should not alter or delay the administration of the induction regimen.

During remission induction, blood counts and necessary blood chemistry analyses should be obtained at least twice weekly — and more often if clinical problems develop or if previous normal values are becoming abnormal.

Repeat bone marrow examination should be performed after 2 and again after 4 weeks to assess the progress of treatment. If no or very little leukemic cell reduction has taken place by these times, consideration should be given to switching to the more rigorous regimen used to induce remission in AML (see below).

Extramedullary ALL will usually respond somewhat to systemic chemotherapy so that it is rarely necessary to add local therapy (e. g., radiation, intrathecal chemotherapy) at this stage. Although CNS leukemia is not eradicated by remission induction drugs, intrathecal methotrexate has proven excessively toxic to adults when given together with vincristine and daunorubicin. Accordingly, it is better reserved until remission has been achieved. If overt symptoms of meningeal leukemia, cranial nerve palsies, and/or communicating hydrocephalus occur, then small (200–400 rad) fractions of total cranial vault radiation should be added to the induction regimen followed by a full CNS treatment regimen as soon as bone marrow remission has been secured.

Remission Maintenance

Achieving a complete remission is only the first, though essential, step in the attempt to cure the disease. In all cases treatment to the body as a whole, plus the central nervous system, must be delivered during remission.

For "common" ALL this treatment should consist of methotrexate and 6-mercaptopurine, given first intensively, then by a continuous, moderate dose schedule. A standard regimen consists of two courses of 6-mercaptopurine 500 mg/m^2 i. v. plus methotrexate 15 mg/m^2 i. v. on days 1-5, given 2 weeks apart. As these courses may produce leukopenia and thrombocytopenia, the cotrimoxazole adjunctive therapy used during remission induction should be continued. Since both drugs are excreted by the kidneys, a creatinine clearance of more than 60 ml/min is required. If the clearance is 30–60 ml/min, the doses of both antimetabolites should be reduced to 50 %. If the creatinine clearance is less than 30 ml/min, this "consolidation" treatment should be withheld. In addition to creatinine clearance, measurements of serum SGOT and bilirubin and a complete blood count should be performed before each course. Treatment should be delayed if any significant abnormalities are present, e. g., bilirubin >3.0 mg/100 ml, SGOT >300, granulocytes $>1500/\mu l$, platelets $<100\,000\ \mu l$.

At the completion of the two intensive courses, all patients should next receive central nervous system treatment. This can take several forms; one which takes about 2 weeks combines high energy radiation therapy to the entire calvarium to the level of C2 with five intrathecal doses of methotrexate or combined drugs [methotrexate, cytosine arabinaside (Ara-C), hydrocortisone]. Radiation should be administered in 12 equal fractions of 200 rads with shielding of the lenses of the eye to prevent cataract formation. Drugs should be given by lumbar puncture, dissolved in 10 ml normal saline, sterile water, or Elliot's B solution (an artificial spinal fluid). The drugs should consist of methotrexate 10 mg and 50 mg each of hydrocortisone and Ara-C. Alternatively, the same combination can be given for 8 weeks during the consolidation therapy (a total of three doses) and subsequently at 8-week intervals for as long as methotrexate and 6-mercaptopurine are given for maintenance (see below).

For B and T cell ALL, in addition to the above measures the patient should receive additional consolidation courses consisting of (a) a course of Ara-C/daunorubicin similar to that given for AML, i. e.., 7 days of Ara-C, 100 mg/m^2 q 12 h subcutaneously plus daunorubicin 45 mg/m^2 i. v. on days 1 and 2 followed by (b) a course of Ara-C 100 mg/m^2 q 12 h for 4 days together with cyclophosphamide 650 mg/m^2 i. v. on the first day. These courses should be reinstituted every 4 months during 4- to 6-week periods in which maintenance methotrexate and 6-mercaptopurine (see below) are interrupted. Patients should be placed on prophylactic cotrimoxazole orally during each of these periods, and weekly complete blood counts obtained, since significant myelosuppression can be anticipated to follow each intensive course.

Following the *consolidation* therapy, intensive chemotherapy courses plus CNS treatment, and recovery from myelosuppression, continual low dose *maintenance* therapy should be employed for a minimum of 2 additional years. An extensively evaluated maintenance regimen consists of methotrexate 25 mg/m^2 p. o. weekly plus 6-mercaptopurine 90 mg/m^2 p. o. daily. Blood counts should be obtained every 2 weeks initially, and then once a month (minimum), adjusting the dosage of antimetabolites so as to maintain blood granulocytes above 1000/µl and platelets above 100 000/µl. Allopurinol and trimethoprim-sulfamethoxazole (Septra or Bactrim) need not be continued during this program.

About one-quarter of complete remitters with common ALL will survive in remission indefinitely. Those with T and B cell leukemia have a much worse prognosis. All individuals with the latter forms of ALL should be considered for allogeneic bone marrow grafting provided (a) they are under 40 years of age and (b) a suitable donor, i. e., a healthy, willing, HLA-matched sibling, is available. Patients with common ALL should be treated with drugs alone. Those who relapse can be returned to remission in more than 50% of cases, and marrow grafting can then be attempted at a transplant center.

Remission Reinduction

Remission reinduction regimens include, in rough order of preference:

1. Vincristine, prednisone, daunorubicin, and asparaginase — as described above. Allergic reactions to *E. coli* L-asparaginase (the conventional form) are common, and *Erwinia* asparaginase may need to be substituted.
2. Ara-C plus daunorubicin given in the manner described below for the treatment of AML.
3. Methotrexate plus asparaginase. Methotrexate is given as a single infusion at 7- to 10-day intervals at increasing doses, each dose being followed 24 h by a single dose of asparaginase 5000 Iµ/m^2. The starting dose of methotrexate is 30 mg/m^2, escalated at 30 mg/m^2 increments to as high as 200 mg/m^2. Careful monitoring of renal function is essential and methotrexate reduction for low creatinine clearance must be made as earlier described in the section on remission consolidation.
4. Cytosine arabinoside plus asparaginase, as described below for the treatment of AML.

Remission maintenance can be similar to that used earlier during the first remission of ALL or the first remission of AML, or can take the form of the regimens used for the treatment of non-Hodgkin's lymphomas, e. g., CHOP or COP. As noted above, young adults with HLA-matched donors should be sent to a transplant center for bone marrow grafting.

Acute Myeloid Leukemia

Remission Induction

The basis for treatment of more resistant leukemias is the combination of an anthracycline and Ara-C. Many other combinations, as well as high dose daunorubicin or high dose Ara-C, have been employed alone with no greater success. Successful treatment demands marked cytoreduction, almost always approaching marrow aplasia. The more rapidly this is accomplished, the quicker normal hematopoiesis will be achieved. Failure to achieve rapid leukemic cell reduction signals a need for a modification of treatment; thus close monitoring of the bone marrow is essential.

Initial treatment should consist of daunorubicin 45 mg/m^2 daily for three successive days by careful intravenous injection or infusion together with a continuous intravenous infusion of Ara-C, 100 mg/m^2 daily, for 7 days. A bone marrow aspiration and biopsy should be performed on the 6th day of treatment. If hypoplasia coupled with reduction of myeloblasts to less than 30% is not achieved, treatment with Ara-C should be continued for three additional days. Treatment should be temporarily interrupted after the first course, save for necessary supportive care, and the bone marrow monitored at weekly intervals. If, after 3 weeks, repopulation with normal cells has not begun, and leukemic myeloblasts persist, a second course of daunorubicin and Ara-C should be tried. A word of caution is necessary. It may be difficult on any one marrow to distinguish residual leukemic from normal regenerating myeloblasts. When in doubt, it is important to wait for 4–7 days, and then to repeat the bone marrow examination. Malignant myeloblastic infiltrates will persist or increase during this interval, signaling the need for further treatment. In recovering marrow, the myeloblasts will decrease and more mature elements will appear through maturation, indicating that further treatment can be deferred until peripheral blood counts are restored to normal. Overall, about 40%–50% of patients will remit after one course of daunorubicin and Ara-C, another 20%–30% will remit after a second course, and the remaining 20%–40% will fail to respond to this regimen.

Once in remission, with bone marrow function restored and drug side effects healed, the same combination of drugs, Ara-C and daunorubicin, given as a 5-day course, should be alternated at 1-month intervals with Ara-C plus 6-thioguanine, and Ara-C plus cyclophosphamide. The doses, schedules, and routes of administration are as follows:

All courses: Ara-C 100 mg q 12 h subcutaneously daily for 5 days
Courses 1, 4, 7, etc.:   daunorubicin 45 mg/m^2 on day 1 (discontinue when a total of 450 m g/m^2 has been accumulated)
Courses 2, 5, 8, etc.:   6-thioguanine 100 mg/m^2 daily for 5 days
Courses 3, 6, 9, etc.:   cyclophosphamide 100 mg/m^2 daily for 5 days

Administration of the courses should continue until relapse or for 3 years. It should be emphasized that the intensity and duration of maintenance treatment is currently under investigation, and the above recommendations will doubtless change.

Meningeal leukemia in adults with AML is uncommon (occurring in about 7% of cases overall). This is in striking contrast to its frequency in ALL and pediatric age AML. Therefore, a lumbar puncture should be performed once a month or so into remission, and treatment initiated only if leukemia cells are identified. Whenever possible the spinal fluid analysis should include examination of cell concentrates prepared with a cytocentrifuge. If the examination is negative, treatment to the CNS can be delayed until signs and symptoms do occur later. The one major exception to this course of expectant management is with acute monocytic leukemia (M_6). With this subtype, meningeal involvement is common enough to warrant prophylactic treatment comparable to that used in ALL (see p. 24).

The standard treatment of AML described above is appropriate for all adult patients up to 70 years of age, and for those under 40 years of age without an HLA identical sibling. For older patients, the dosage of daunorubicin should be reduced to 30 mg/m^2 per dose. Patients in their twenties or thirties with a suitable donor should be treated to remission as outlined, and then referred to a bone marrow transplantation center for allogeneic bone marrow engraftment. The risks of transplantation in older patients, or those with mismatched donors, are so uniformly grave that transplantation should not be considered.

Treatment of Relapse

Treatment at relapse is always more uncertain than at first presentation. However, the same general principles apply, i. e., rapid and extensive cytoreduction and scrupulous supportive care. The complete remission rate varies from 25% to 50%, and remission duration, with or without remission maintenance, averages about 6 months. Remission induction regimens include Ara-C plus daunorubicin as used in primary treatment, Ara-C plus thioguanine, POMP (prednisone 250–1000 mg/m^2 i. v. daily × 5 days, vincristine 2 mg i. v. on day 1, methotrexate 7.5 mg/m^2 daily × 5 days, plus 6-mercaptopurine 500 mg/m^2 daily × 5 days), or high dose Ara-C with or without L-asparaginase. The latter program involves sequential treatment with 2–3 g Ara-C given by contionuous 3-h infusions q 12 h for a total of four doses, followed by L-asparaginase 6000 units/m^2 i. m. 3 h after the end of the fourth and last Ara-C infusion. This regimen is repeated every week until remission is achieved. This latter regimen is effective but toxicity, especially conjunctivities, gastrointestinal complaints, and cerebellar symptoms and signs, is common. Conjunctivitis can be ameliorated by the frequent use of eyewashes. The patient should also be required to write his name daily, and with the first sign of major deterioration in handwriting, Ara-C treatment should be discontinued. With failure to respond to the above regimens the patient faces the alternatives only of experimental therapy or supportive care alone.

Complications of Therapy

Complications during therapy are usually the result of one of two factors: injury to organs as a side effect of the drugs employed, and the heightened release of toxic products of cell lysis resulting from therapy. The latter has already been covered in the discussion of induction and is rarely a problem after the first 1–2 weeks of treatment. Of drug side effects, the most prominent and threatening are myelosuppression and immunosuppression, and the resultant increases in hemorrhage and infection.

Bleeding because of thrombocytopenia is treated with platelet transfusions. Platelets should be given whenever the platelet count falls below 20 000/µl or when severe bleeding occurs as a result of local injury or ulceration in patients with platelet counts of less than 80 000/µl. Febrile patients with thrombocytopenia are particularly prone to spontaneous bleeding; indeed, bleeding is uncommon in afebrile patients, even those with severe thrombocytopenia.

Infections associated with severe granulopenia are usually caused by gram-negative bacilli, *Klebsiella, Aerobacter, Proteus,* and *Pseudomonas* species, *E. coli* and *Staphylococcus aureus.* As visceral infections frequently cannot be documented on initial cultures, and can be rapidly lethal, fever (> 38.5 °C) of unknown etiology occurring in granulocytopenic patients should be treated by an antibiotic combination which provides coverage for the common gram-positive and gram-negative organisms. The most extensively tested combinations include an aminoglycoside plus a synthetic penicillin with antipseudomonal activity. Our current preferred combination is mezlocillin $12/m^2$ daily plus tobramycin, 3–5 mg/kg daily, each divided into three doses given every 8 h.

Ticarcillin is a suitable alternative penicillin and gentamicin and amikacin are alternative aminoglycosides. Treatment, when successful in reducing fever and resolving symptoms, should be continued for 10 days or until granulocyte counts have returned to normal. When fever persists for more than 3–5 days and no organism has been cultured, the most common problem is either a fungal superinfection or, in patients with indwelling Hickmann or Broviak catheters, a superinfection with *Streptococcus viridans* or *Staphylococcus epidermidis.* A careful search for areas of infection should be undertaken, including urine, sputum, and bone marrow cultures for fungi, and catheter blood as well as venous blood from points distant from the catheter site should be cultured. If there is clinical evidence of a catheter infection or if *Staph. epidermidis* or *Strep. viridans* is cultured, vancomycin is added at a dose of 1–1.5 g by 30-min infusion every 12 h and the original antibiotics should be continued. If no organism is discovered in a persistently febrile patient or if fungi are cultured from blood, marrow, or urine, amphotericin B should be added. A 1 mg test dose should be given intravenously after 2 h and the patient observed for bronchospasm and hypotension. If none occurs, an initial dose of 25 mg should be given, followed by 0.5–1.0 mg/kg daily until a response is achieved *and* a total of 1–2 g has been given.

With the administration of these antibiotics, and especially with aminoglycosides, vancomycin, and amphotericin B, renal function and electrolyte balance should be carefully monitored and dose reductions made as appropriate.

Once the remission maintenance phase is reached, immunosuppression becomes the most serious complication and infections caused by *Pneumocystis carinii,* cytomegalovirus, Legionella, and the like become predominant. Fever, nonproductive cough, and dyspnea should be evaluated without delay if pneumocystitis is suspected, and all cytotoxic drugs should be discontinued and the patient started immediately on cotrimoxazole (Bactrim, Septra).

Cotrimoxazole as a prophylactic should be administered to patients receiving intensive remission induction and remission consolidation therapy and continued through the period of granulocytopenia. It should be given as two tablets t. i. d. orally. This adjunct does not need to be continued during remission maintenance, any infections being treated appropriately as they arise.

Psychologically, as well as physically, acute leukemia is a devastating illnes. The diagnosis is considered a death sentence by most patients, and indeed that assessment is warranted all too often. However, in a fortunate minority death is avoided or forestalled for many months and years, and life can be productive and happy. This positive aspect, and the availability of effective treatments, should be stressed, so that the quality of whatever measure of life that can be gained is maximized.

The most important aspects of support depend upon developing a relationship of trust between the patient and the medical team. With rare exceptions all aspects of care should be discussed, being careful to let the patient control the scope of the discussion. Answers to questions should be accurate but should stress the positive aspects of care and prognosis. Every patient should be cautioned about overextending himself — physically, emotionally, economically, etc. — but within reasonable limits encouraged to live life as fully as possible. It should be emphasized that during remission there are few limits that need to be placed on any of the normal activities of the patient.

Further Reading

Bennett JM, Catovsky D, Daniel MT, Flandrin G, Galton DAG, Galnick HR, Sultan C, The French-American British (FAB) Cooperative Group (1981) The morphological classification of acute lymphoblastic leukemia: concordance among observers and clinical correlations. Br J Haematol. 47: 553–561

Bennett JM, Catovsky D, Daniel MT, Flandrin G, Galton DAG, Galnick HR, Sultan C, The French-American British (FAB) Cooperative Group (1985) Proposed revised criteria for the classification of acute myeloid leukemia. Ann Intern Med 103: 629–629

Henderson ES (1969) Treatment of acute leukemia. In: Holland JF Jr., Miescher PA, Jaffe ER (eds) Leukemia and lymphoma. Grune and Stratton, New York pp 47–95

Editorial Comment

The FAB (French–American–British) classification, first introduced in 1976, has gained wide acceptance because it has provided a common language for physicians and scientists. Not only has the classification led to meaningful comparison of treatment results, but it also has prognostic significance for remission induction and survival. For ALL the members of the FAB group had a concordance between seven observers of 63%. In 1980, the group introduced a simplified scoring system for types L_1 and L_2 and the overall concordance increased to 84%. L_3 has not changed.

The original description of four types of acute myeloid leukemia led to difficulties. Experts from the Southwest Oncology Group found the FAB classification reproducible in only 70% of instances, and even the members of the FAB group had major disagreements when reviewing 71 preselected bone marrows. All seven members agreed in only 26 cases; 6 agreed in 17 cases, 5 in 17 cases, and 4 in 11 cases. The group has proposed new criteria (recently published in the Annals of Internal Medicine), and improved its overall concordance from 60% to 82%.

The new criteria appear to improve the classification, but problems remain. Ever since bone marrows were first aspirated, hematologists have had little difficulty in recognizing the distinctive features of acute promyelocytic leukemia (M_3) and acute monocytic leukemia (M_5). The requirement of at least 30% myeloblasts, and/or monoblasts is not necessary for these subtypes. But where would one place the marrow containing 30%–40% erythroblasts? Will hematologists at large reach anywhere near the 80% plus concordance obtained by a group of specialists who have met several times since 1976?

The morphology of the bone marrow often presents an opportunity for disagreement among reviewers, just as viewers of modern art can disagree. Even the best classifications, when based on morphology alone, will meet with difficulties, and we are waiting for improved technology in cytogenetics, immunology, and yet to be discovered areas to solve some of the current problems.

3. Myeloproliferative Disorders:
Polycythemia Vera, Essential Thrombocythemia, and Idiopathic Myelofibrosis/Agnogenic Myeloid Metaplasia

H. J. Iland and J. Laszlo

Introduction

In 1951 William Dameshek speculated that under certain conditions hematopoietic cells (precursors of erythrocytes, granulocytes, and platelets), as well as fibroblasts, proliferated "en masse" within the bone marrow in response to a myelostimulatory factor. This factor, said Dameshek, appeared also to activate dormant embryonal hematopoietic tissue in the liver and spleen. These processes resulted in a spectrum of clinicopathologic entities which Dameshek referred to as the myeloproliferative syndromes. The concept of myeloproliferative syndrome, which was well grounded in studies of hematopathology by earlier workers, has gained widespread acceptance, although more recent knowledge about hematopoiesis has necessitated certain modifications to the original hypothesis.

Excessive proliferation of one or more hematopoietic elements is the hallmark of myeloproliferative disorders (MPDs), among which both acute and chronic subgroups are

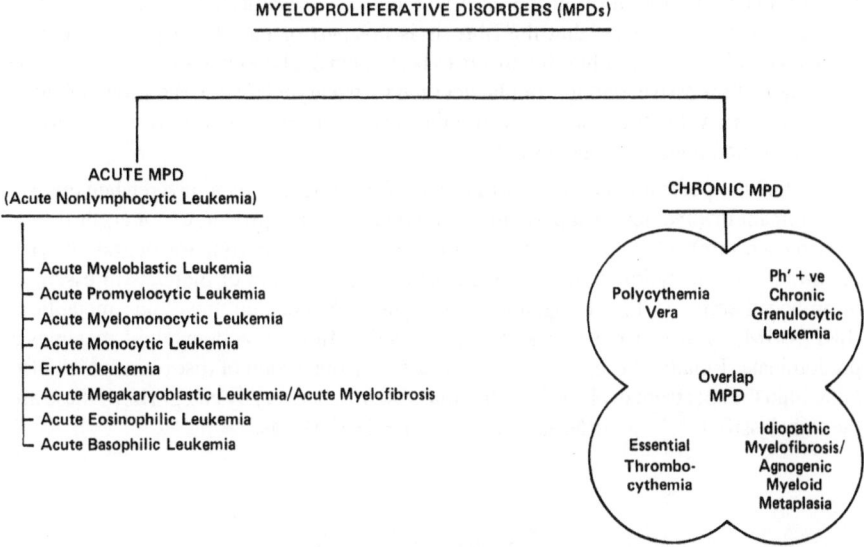

Fig. 1. The spectrum of acute and chronic myeloproliferative disorders

recognized (Fig. 1). The former include all the variants of acute nonlymphocytic leukemia, which are characterized by excessive proliferation of primitive cells with marked impairment of maturation. Abnormal proliferation is also a feature of chronic MPDs, but maturation is less severely affected.

The clonal, and therefore neoplastic, nature of MPDs has been clearly demonstrated by cytogenetic analyses, isoenzyme studies of glucose-6-phosphate dehydrogenase heterozygotes, and clonogenic asays. In addition, these studies indicate that in most cases the target of the neoplastic transformation is the hematopoietic stem cell, a progenitor committed to the myeloid pathway of differentiation (i. e., to granulocytes, monocytes, erythrocytes, and platelets). In lymphoid blast crisis of chronic granulocytic leukemia however, the neoplastic cell is capable of both myeloid and lymphoid differentiation and sometimes exhibits features of both cell types simultaneously. Since its potential for differentiation is less restricted than that of the hematopoietic stem cell, it represents a more primitive progenitor within the stem cell hierarchy — the putative lymphohematopoietic pluripotent stem cell. In contrast, in some cases of acute nonlymphocytic leukemia the neoplastic process involves only granulocytes and monocytes; the neoplastic cell is committed to a more restricted pathway of differentiation and is therefore less primitive than the hematopoietic stem cell. Regardless of the type of stem cell involved, the result is impairment of the normal regulatory mechanisms governing self-renewal, proliferation, differentiation, and maturation.

Since the acute leukemias are dealt with in Chapter 2, the remainder of this review will be confined to chronic MPDs. These conditions exhibit the following characteristics, to varying extents:

1. Panhyperplasia of hematopoietic elements within the bone marrow (erythrocytic, granulocytic ± monocytic, and megakaryocytic)
2. Extramedullary hematopoiesis (myeloid metaplasia) in the spleen and, to a lesser extent, in the liver and other tissues
3. Fibroblastic proliferation in the marrow [contrary to Dameshek's postulate, available evidence indicates that the fibrosis is not part of the clonal proliferation of hematopoietic cells; rather, it appears to be a reactive phenomenon, possibly due to release of excessive amounts of platelet (and megakaryocyte) derived growth factor]
4. A propensity for transformation to either acute leukemia or progressive marrow fibrosis and myeloid metaplasia

Within the spectrum of chronic MPDs, specific entities are recognized when there is predominant involvement of a particular cell type. Thus overproduction of erythrocytes is the most prominent feature in polycythemia vera (PV), overproduction of granulocytes in chronic granulocytic leukemia (CGL), and overproduction of platelets in essential thrombocythemia (ET). Idiopathic myelofibrosis/agnogenic myeloid metaplasia (IMF/AMM) is also a chronic MPD, but reactive fibrosis and myeloid metaplasia predominate. Finally, there is a large and heterogeneous group of disorders which also fall within the spectrum of chronic MPDs but which are less easily categorized; these are the "unclassifiable," "undifferentiated", or "overlap" MPDs.

Polycythemia Vera

Polycythemia vera (PV) is the preferred term, but this condition has also been called polycythemia rubra vera, primary polycythemia, erythremia, splenomegalic polycythemia, and Vaquez-Osler disease.

Although PV exhibits all the features of chronic MPDs to some extent, its predominant manifestation is accelerated erythropoiesis which results in excessive red cell production and an absolute erythrocytosis (i. e., an increased total red blood cell mass). At the time of initial presentation the degree of extramedullary hematopoiesis is usually mild, and marrow fibrosis is minimal or absent. However, a "spent" phase gradually supervenes in 15%–20% of patients. This stage of the disease is also known as burned-out polycythemia or postpolycythemic myeloid metaplasia; it is virtually indistinguishable from the idiopathic variety (IMF/AMM).

Epidemiology

Polycythemia vera is a relatively uncommon disorder with an annual incidence of less than ten new case per million. Males are affected only slightly more often than females; the median age at diagnosis is approximately 60 years, with the majority of patients being at least 45 years of age. The etiology is unknown.

Symptoms and Signs

The disease has an insidious onset and the diagnosis may be suggested only by finding an elevated hemoglobin (Hb) or hematocrit (Hct) in an apparently healthy person. On the other hand, development of a variety of complications may precipitate recognition of the disease.

Expansion of the red cell mass is associated with hyperviscosity, which in turn causes circulatory disturbances in many organs. Thus headaches, dizziness, visual phenomena (blurred vision, diplopia, scotomata) and tinnitus are common cerebral manifestations. Similarly, erythromelalgia (painful red extremities), paresthesias and burning sensations, particularly in the feet, intermittent claudication, myocardial ischemia, and mesenteric ischemia reflect impairment of blood supply to the peripheral circulation, the heart, and the gut, respectively. Venous thromboembolism may occur, and a hemorrhagic diathesis is also seen. The mucous membranes and skin are occasional sites of blood loss, while life-threatening hemorrhage may occur in association with surgery, trauma, or a peptic ulcer. Fever, night sweats, and weight loss may occur as a result of a hypermetabolic state; gouty arthritis, uric acid calculi, or urate nephropathy occur in 5%–10% of patients because of increased uric acid production as a consequence of accelerated nucleic acid turnover.

Splenomegaly is present in about 75% of patients at the time of initial presentation. Splenic enlargement is usually mild to moderate, and it may be responsible for early satiety, abdominal fullness, and left hypochondrial pain. Pruritus, especially after a warm bath, is a common symptom; together with urticaria and peptic ulcers, this appears to be related to increased histamine production by basophils and other granulocytes.

Other manifestations include hypertension, facial plethora with conjunctival and mucosal congestion, and distension of retinal veins.

The Spent Phase

The median duration from the time of diagnosis of PV to the onset of postpolycythemic myeloid metaplasia (PPMM) is approximately 10 years. A reduction in the intensity of therapy necessary for control of erythrocytosis may be the earliest sign of this stage of the disease (see p. 40). As the process continues, the Hb, Hct, and red cell mass stabilize, and eventually anemia may develop; bleeding and splenomegaly also become more troublesome. Progressive hepatomegaly may occur, and portal hypertension and ascites are being increasingly recognized.

Differential Diagnosis

Chronic MPDs form a spectrum of conditions which at times are difficult to distinguish from each other. In particular, PV may be confused with ET since blood loss and iron deficiency can mask the erythrocytosis of PV and even aggravate any preexisting thrombocytosis. Cautious replacement of iron stores is the only reliable way to establish a definitive diagnosis in this situation: only in PV will the Hb, Hct, and red cell mass rise to polycythemic levels.

Overt PV must also be distinguished from the many causes of secondary polycythemia and from relative polycythemia (Table 1). In many cases, this can be done on the basis of a history and physical examination, but in other cases, a sequence of investigations may be necessary.

Diagnostic Approach

Suspicion of PV should be aroused in the following situations: (a) any time a patient manifests the symptoms or signs described above; (b) the finding of an elevated Hb or Hct; (c) the finding of a normal Hb or Hct despite the presence of significant iron deficiency. The importance of a diagnostic iron trial has already been mentioned. Subsequent investigations should be directed at answering three key questions, discussed individually below.

Is the Erythrocytosis Absolute or Relative?

Relative polycythemia occurs whenever there is an elevated Hb or Hct in the absence of an absolute increase in the total red cell mass; it is due to an increase in the ratio of the red cell mass to the plasma volume. This can occur as a result of dehydration, but the commonest cause of a chronically elevated Hct is Gaisböck's syndrome (also known as stress polycythemia or pseudopolycythemia). A subgroup of patients with Gaisböck's

Table 1. Classification of erythrocytosis

I.   *Polycythemia vera*

II. *Secondary polycythemia*
     A. Physiologically appropriate increase in erythropoietin

     1. High altitude
     2. Intrathoracic shunt (right to left)
        (a) Cyanotic congenital heart disease
        (b) Cirrhosis
        (c) Hereditary hemorrhagic telangiectasia
        (d) Other pulmonary arteriovenous malformations
     3. Chronic respiratory disease
     4. Alveolar hypoventilation (obesity/somnolence syndrome, Pickwickian syndrome)
     5. Defective oxygen transport
        (a) Smoking (carbon monoxide)
        (b) High oxygen affinity hemoglobinopathy
        (c) Congenital reduction in red cell 2,3-diphosphoglycerate
     6. Defective oxidative metabolism (cobalt therapy)

     B. Physiologically inappropriate increase in erythropoietin
     1. Renal disorders
        (a) Renal artery stenosis
        (b) Renal transplant rejection
        (c) Cyst
        (d) Hydronephrosis
        (e) Renal tumors
     2. Endocrine disorders
        (a) Pheochromocytoma
        (b) Conn's syndrome
        (c) Cushing's syndrome
        (d) Androgen-secreting ovarian tumors
     3. Other tumors
        (a) Uterine fibroids
        (b) Cerebellar hemangioblastoma
        (c) Hepatoma
     4. Hereditary autonomous overproduction of erythropoietin

III. *Relative polycythemia*
     A. Stress polycythemia (pseudopolycythemia, Gaisböck's syndrome)
     B. Dehydration

---

syndrome tend to be obese, hypertensive, anxious males who smoke heavily and have an increased incidence of thromboembolic and cardiovascular disease. It remains unclear whether the high Hct is responsible for the increased morbidity and shortened life expectancy of these patients. Since myelosuppression is an inappropriate therapy for such individuals, it is essential to distinguish accurately between relative and absolute polycythemia. The most reliable method involves determination of the total red blood cell mass (utilizing the patient's [51]chromium-labeled red cells) and the plasma volume (with [125]iodine-labeled albumin). Absolute erythrocytosis is present when the total red blood

35

cell mass is $\geqslant 36$ ml/kg in males and $\geqslant 32$ ml/kg in females. If reliable radioisotope testing is not available, even greater reliance must be placed on the investigations described below.

Is There Any Evidence Directly Supporting a Diagnosis of Polycythemia Vera?

Peripheral Blood. Elevation of the Hb and Hct are the most important findings; however, masked polycythemia may be present with a normal Hb and Hct if there is also evidence of iron deficiency such as microcytosis, hypochromia, and polychromasia (reticulocytosis). Moderate leukocytosis (due predominantly to neutrophilia with or without basophilia, eosinophilia, and occasional circulating myeloid precursors) and thrombocytosis (with or without morphologically abnormal forms) may also be present. The white cell count is usually less than $50\,000/\mu l$ (in contrast to CGL), and the platelet count is usually less than $1\,000\,000/\mu l$ (in contrast to ET). The erythrocyte sedimentation rate is characteristically low in PV (<1 mm/h Westergren).

As the spent phase develops, red cell morphology becomes progressively more abnormal (anisocytosis and poikilocytosis with prominent teardrop cells), and a leukoerythroblastic picture appears (increasing numbers of circulating myeloid and erythroid precursors). The white cell and platelet counts may rise further or fall to abnormally low levels.

Bone Marrow. Ideally both an aspirate and a biopsy should be obtained; cellular morphology and iron content are best appreciated with the former, while the latter provides the best assessment of cellularity and content of reticulin and collagen. The most important reason for sampling the bone marrow is to confirm that a myeloproliferative process is

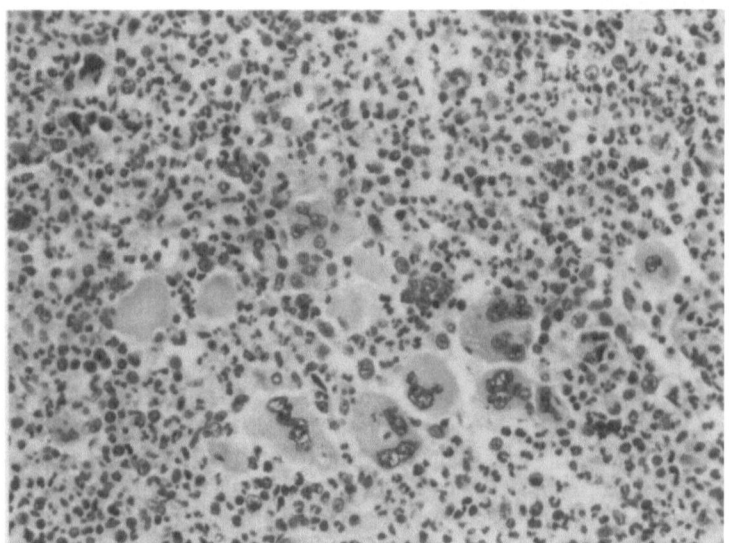

Fig. 2. Hypercellular bone marrow in the erythrocytotic phase of PV (by courtesy of Dr. Powers Peterson, Polycythemia Vera Study Group). ×325

indeed present; because of the overlap with other MPDs a specific diagnosis of PV cannot always be established.

The majority of patients with untreated PV will have significant marrow hypercellularity ($\geqslant 60\%$ of the cross-sectional area of the biopsy, see Fig. 2). This is due to a pan-hyperplasia (increased erythroid, myeloid, and megakaryocytic elements), in contrast to secondary polycythemia, in which hyperplasia is usually confined to the erythroid series. The megakaryocytes are often increased in size as well as in number. Iron stores, as demonstrated by Prussian blue staining, are deficient in the vast majority of patients; this probably reflects increased utilization of iron by the expanded erythroid mass, or it may be due to occult blood loss. The reticulin content (as demonstrated by a Foot and Foot silver impregnation stain), is normal or only slightly increased in approximately 90% of patients prior to treatment.

Serial bone marrow biopsies may show increasing deposition of reticulin as the spent phase develops (Fig. 3), and collagen fibrosis (azan trichrome stain) also becomes apparent. Cellularity usually decreases, although megakaryocytosis may persist.

Spleen Size. Splenomegaly is a frequent finding in PV (and other MPDs); however, unless the spleen is enlarged to at least twice the normal size, it may not be palpable. In the absence of facilities for radioisotopic imaging of the spleen, an estimate of spleen size can be obtained by plain X-radiography of the upper abdomen.

Leukocyte Alkaline Phosphatase. When a peripheral blood film is stained for leukocyte alkaline phosphatase (LAP), an LAP score can be obtained by grading the enzyme activity in each of 100 neutrophils from 0 to 4 and then summing the individual values obtained. The LAP score is elevated in the majority of patients with PV; in secondary polycythemia it is usually normal (in the absence of infection, inflammation, or hormonal therapy).

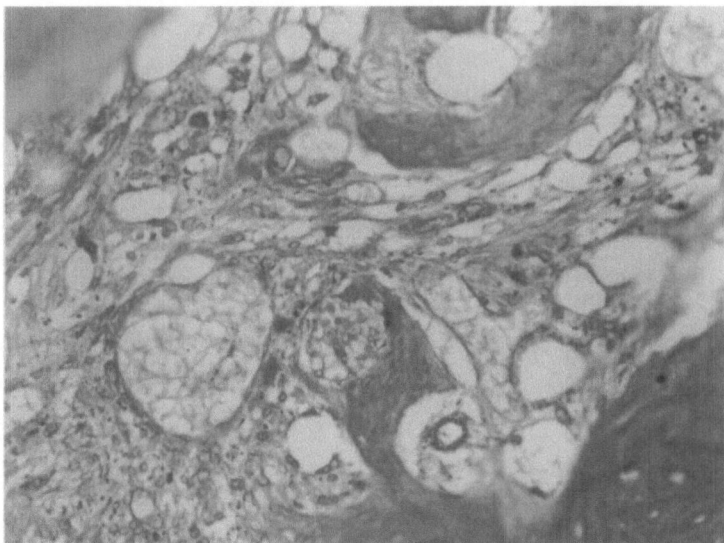

Fig. 3. Silver impregnation stain in the spent phase of PV showing increased reticulin deposition (by courtesy of Dr. Powers Peterson, Polycythemia Vera Study Group). ×250

37

Since the upper limit of normal (approximately 100) varies somewhat from institution to institution, it is essential that a normal control sample be assayed concurrently to ensure accurate interpretation.

Biochemical Findings. Several biochemical studies are helpful, though not essential, in establishing a diagnosis of PV. The serum vitamin B_{12} level and the unbound B_{12} binding capacity ($UB_{12}BC$) are frequently elevated in PV and other MPDs, because of elevated levels of B_{12} binding proteins in serum and leukocytes (transcobalamins I and III). Elevated levels of uric acid, bilirubin, histamine, and lysozyme are found in many patients. Staining the marrow for iron is a more reliable means of assessing iron stores than is measurement of the serum iron and total iron binding capacity.

Miscellaneous. Platelet function studies and cytogenetics may yield abnormal results in patients with PV, but they are not specific enough to be diagnostically useful. Erythropoietin assays in plasma and urine are helpful in distinguishing PV from secondary polycythemia when no cause for the latter can be found; in PV, erythropoietin is decreased or absent, while the level is increased in secondary polycythemia.

Can Secondary Causes of Erythrocytosis Be Excluded?

Since there are many causes of secondary polycythemia (Table 1), an attempt should be made to exclude at least the most frequent offenders. A chest-X-ray is a useful adjunct to physical examination for detection of chronic respiratory disease, cardiac disease, or large pulmonary arteriovenous malformations. Measurement of arterial oxygen saturation (S_aO_2) should be performed whenever possible, to exclude arterial hypoxemia as a cause of secondary polycythemia. The S_aO_2 should be $\geqslant 92\%$ in PV; levels below 88% are strongly suggestive of secondary polycythemia due to hypoxemia. Similarly, carboxy-Hb normally constitutes $<1.5\%$ of total Hb, but in erythrocytosis caused by heavy smoking the proportion of carboxy-Hb is usually $>6\%$.

Table 2. PVSG criteria for polycythemia vera

Category A	Category B

1. Increased red cell mass
   Male $\geqslant 36$ ml/kg
   Female $\geqslant 32$ ml/kg
	1. Thrombocytosis
	   Platelets $>400\,000/\mu l$

2. Normal arterial O_2 saturation
   $S_aO_2 \geqslant 92\%$
	2. Leukocytosis
	   White cells $>12\,000/\mu l$

3. Splenomegaly	3. Elevated LAP score >100 (no fever or infection)

	4. Elevated serum vitamin
	   $B_{12} >900$ pg/ml
	   or $UB_{12}BC >2200$ pg/ml

Patients are regarded as having PV if either of the following combinations is present:

A1+A2+A3

or

A1+A2+any two parameters from category B

A vast array of renal disorders can also cause secondary polycythemia, and intravenous pyelography should therefore be inluded in the evaluation of all patients with suspected PV.

PVSG Criteria

Since no single test can unequivocally establish a diagnosis of PV and highly specialized studies may be required to exclude rare causes of secondary polycythemia (e. g., construction of oxygen dissociation curves for detection of hemoglobinopathies), the Polycythemia Vera Study Group (PVSG) in 1968 proposed a set of criteria which indicate a high probability of PV in the absence of recognizable secondary causes. Their sensitivity and specificity are such that they remain the most widely used diagnostic criteria for PV (Table 2).

Prognosis

Modern treatment programs which carefully control erythroid overproduction by means of phlebotomy and/or myelosuppression have resulted in significant increases in median survival, to approximately 10 years (as compared with 18 months in untreated patients). Nevertheless, patients with PV still have a shorter life expectancy than age- and sex-matched controls. The major complications which may limit survival include thrombosis and hemorrhage, leukemic and nonleukemic second malignancies, and PPMM.

Large-scale, long-term randomized studies of treatment options by the PVSG have contributed significantly to our ability to provide optimal, individualized therapy, by demonstrating that the complications of PV are influenced to a large extent by the type of therapy employed.

Major thrombotic phenomena constitute the leading causes of morbidity and mortality in PV, particularly among patients treated by phlebotomy alone. Second malignances appear to occur more commonly in myelosuppressed patients, particularly acute leukemia and gastrointestinal and skin cancers. Retrospective studies suggest that ionizing radiation may be a significant factor in the development of PPMM, but this has not yet been confirmed by prospective studies.

Treatment

The primary aim of therapy during the active (erythrocytotic) phase of PV is to reduce the total red blood cell mass, thereby lowering the whole blood viscosity. Both induction and maintenace programs are involved. Assessment of the venous Hct in a Wintrobe tube is the simplest and most convenient method of evaluating the response to therapy.

Secondary aims, which may not be relevant for all patients, include control of other manifestations of the myeloproliferative state (i. e., thrombocytosis and leukocytosis), reduction of uric acid production and/or excretion, control of intractable pruritus, treatment of the spent phase, and management of postpolycythemic acute leukemia.

Treatment of the Erythrocytotic Phase

Induction. Rapid reduction of the Hct is the most important objective of an induction regimen. Removal of 500 ml blood every 2–3 days is the simplest and safest method of lowering the Hct, which should be reduced to below 45% so as to minimize the risk of thrombohemorrhagic phenomena. In elderly patients or those with preexisting cardiovascular disease, only 250 ml should be removed every 3–4 days. Contraction of the plasma volume by dehydration or diuretic therapy should be avoided, even in patients with congestive cardiac failure, because the resultant increase in whole blood viscosity will negate the effects of venesection.

Maintenance. Once the Hct has been successfully reduced, a long-term program for control of the disease must be instituted. Several options are available and a decision on the optimal approach must be based primarily on individual patient characteristics. Both chronic phlebotomy and myelosuppressive therapy are acceptable alternatives, but both approaches have advantages and disadvantages.

As indicated in the preceding section, manifestations and complications found in patients with PV are related in part to the type of therapy adopted. Since myelosuppression is associated with an increased incidence of postpolycythemic acute leukemia, phlebotomy is the preferred modality in young patients who face many years of treatment. Phlebotomy not only removes red cells from the circulation, but also induces a state of chronic iron deficiency which inhibits Hb synthesis. However, chronic iron deficiency has been associated with a variety of symptoms even when overt anemia is not present. These symptoms include lassitude, irritability, headache, anorexia, glossitis, angular stomatitis, koilonychia, dysphagia, pagophagia (compulsive ice eating, a form of pica), and even pruritus. If these symptoms become too troublesome, myelosuppression should be introduced so that iron replacement therapy can be administered without precipitating overt polycythemia.

The PVSG has demonstrated that long-term treatment by phlebotomy alone is associated with an increased incidence of thrombotic complications such as cerebrovascular accidents, myocardial infarctions, mesenteric ischemia, peripheral arterial occlusions, and venous thromboembolism, particularly during the first few years. Other patients at increased risk of thrombosis are those over 70 years of age and those with a previous history of thrombophlebitis. The addition of platelet anti-aggregating agents (such as aspirin and dipyridamole) to a phlebotomy program does not appear to be consistently effective in preventing thrombosis, and is associated with an increased incidence of gastrointestinal hemorrhage. Thus patients with a high phlebotomy requirement, an age greater than 70, or previous thrombophlebitis should be treated with myelosuppressive agents.

While phlebotomy can control the elevated red blood cell mass, it does not affect the underlying abnormality, i. e., excessive myeloproliferation. Frequent phlebotomy may aggravate thrombocytosis and possibly potentiate the thrombohemorrhagic tendency. Furthermore, symptoms attributable to the hypermetabolic state, to splenomegaly, to increased uric acid production and to abnormal histamine metabolism are not controlled by phlebotomy.

Myelosuppression can be achieved with either chemotherapy or irradiation. Radioactive phosphorus (^{32}P) is the simplest and most efficient method of delivering myelosuppressive radiation. It should be administered intravenously at a dose of 2.3 mCi/m^2 (limit 5 mCi). Responses are relatively slow (several weeks being required for maximal effect), and a second and third dose may be required at intervals of 3 or more months. At least 75% of patients will have a complete response, and in the majority no further therapy is required for 1–2 years. No more than 15 mCi should be given in any 12-month period, and the cumulative dose should not exceed 35 mCi. The side effects of ^{32}P include excessive myelosuppression (rarely a problem if treatment guidelines are adhered to), acute leukemia (in 5%–10% after several years), and nonleukemic second malignancies. ^{32}P therapy can be supplemented with occasional phlebotomies in order to minimize the side effects of both forms of treatment.

A variety of chemotherapeutic agents can be utilized for treatment of PV. The alkylating agents have been the mainstays of chemotherapy in PV and the other MPDs for many years; busulfan and chlorambucil have been used most extensively. The side effects are similar to those seen with ^{32}P, although acute leukemia is even more common and the risks of excessive myelosuppression are also greater. Table 3 summarizes the most commonly employed chemotherapeutic treatment regimens.

The PVSG has now shown that there is a 10%–15% incidence of acute leukemia in patients treated with chlorambucil, and its use is therefore no longer recommended. Busulfan is notorious for its potent stem cell toxicity, and irreversible myelosuppression (particularly thrombocytopenia) is a significant problem. (It should also be noted, however, that unmaintained remissions of many months or even years are sometimes obtained with busulfan.) Other side-effects of busulfan include pulmonary fibrosis, hyperpigmentation, and an Addisonian-like illness. Cyclophosphamide and melphalan can also be employed, although they offer no particular advantages over the more commonly used alkylating agents.

Hydroxyurea, an antimetabolite with little or no oncogenic potential (see Table 3), appears to be as effective as ^{32}P and the alkylating agents, and it has the added advantages that its duration of action is short and it does not appear to exert its effect primarily on stem cells. Side effects include rashes, drug fever, megaloblastoid effects, and my-

Table 3. Chemotherapy in polycythemia vera

Chlorambucil	Initially 10 mg/day for 4 weeks
	Subsequently 2–10 mg/day (higher doses if
	   used intermittently, lower doses if
	   used continuously)

Busulfan	4–6 mg/day intermittently
Melphalan	Initially 6 mg/day for 1 week, then 2–4 mg/day until remission is achieved Maintain with 2 mg 2 or 3 times weekly
Cyclophosphamide	75–150 mg/day intermittently
Hydroxyurea	Initially 15–30 mg/kg daily for 1 week, then 15 mg/kg daily until remission is achieved Maintenance dose dependent upon blood counts

elosuppression that is usually rapidly reversible. The latter can also be a disadvantage in that the period of unmaintained remission tends to be brief.

Surgery poses a serious threat to the polycythemic patient because of the great risk of developing thrombohemorrhagic complications. It is essential that the disease be adequately controlled with myelosuppressive therapy before surgical intervention, especially if splenectomy is contemplated (e. g., during the spent phase), in order to prevent extreme thrombocytosis and the catastrophic consequences which may follow. Since up to 90% of the platelet mass is pooled in a grossly enlarged spleen, splenectomy may result in a precipitous rise in the platelet count, which may be complicated by massive thrombosis or hemorrhage even in a patient without prior history of thrombocytosis.

In summary, therapy should at all times be guided by the predominant manifestations and age of the patient. After initial phlebotomy in all patients, those with relatively mild disease should be given a trial of phlebotomy alone. Patients (a) with more aggressive disease (history of thrombosis, marked constitutional symptoms, or a high phlebotomy requirement), (b) older than 70 years, or (c) undergoing major surgery should be treated with myelosuppressive agents with or without supplemental phlebotomy. We believe that if younger patients require myelosuppression they are best managed with hydroxyurea. In the elderly, either ^{32}P or hydroxyurea is satisfactory; ^{32}P is particularly useful if limited follow-up is likely or whenever patient compliance is a problem.

Adjuvant Therapy in the Erythrocytotic Phase

Uric Acid Overproduction. Hyperuricemia and hyperuricosuria can be prevented by the use of the xanthine oxidase inhibitor allopurinol (300 mg/day). Allopurinol therapy should commence as soon as the diagnosis is established and continue as long as there is evidence of active disease. In patients who receive myelosuppressive therapy, allopurinol can usually be discontinued within several weeks; in patients treated by phlebotomy alone, allopurinol may need to be continued indefinitely.

Pruritus. This distressing symptom is best managed by control of the erythrocytosis. If pruritus persists despite adequate control of erythrocytosis, histamine H_1-receptor antagonists (e. g., cyproheptadine 4–20 mg/day) and H_2-receptor antagonists (e. g., cimetidine 1200 mg/day), either alone or in combination, may be helpful. Some benefit has also been reported with cholestyramine (8–12 g/day), an anion exchange resin that binds bile acids. Ultimately, myelosuppression may be required in refractory cases even though phlebotomy successfully controls the erythrocytosis.

Treatment During the Spent Phase

Once PPMM develops, the prognosis is poor; median survival is of the order of 2 years. Therapy is directed primarily at ameliorating symptoms and has little impact on survival. Since approaches to the management of PPMM and IMF/AMM are essentially identical, the reader is referred to the section dealing with the treatment of IMF/AMM.

Management of Postpolycythemic Acute Leukemia

This complication is almost universally fatal. Treatment is essentially the same as that for de novo acute leukemia. In most instances the acute transformation is myeloid in type, and therapy with daunorubicin and cytosine arabinoside offers the best chance for a response. However, complete remission is infrequently achieved, and survival is measured in weeks to months.

Sometimes the transition to acute leukemia is gradual, with a prolonged preleukemic state characterized by varying combinations of cytopenias and a small number of circulating blast cells. It is probably counterproductive to treat such patients with aggressive leukemia induction regimens. A therapeutic alternative that is being actively studied involves the use of very low doses of cytosine arabinoside and other agents which are capable of inducing differentiation.

Essential Thrombocythemia

Essential thrombocythemia (ET) is also known as hemorrhagic thrombocythemia, primary thrombocythemia, and primary thrombocytosis.

Essential thrombocythemia was the last of the chronic MPDs to be recognized as a discrete entity. This is because marked thrombocytosis, the sine qua non of ET, is also frequently present in PV, CGL, and IMF/AMM. Furthermore, the major clinical and pathologic manifestations of ET (i. e., thromboembolic and hemorrhagic phenomena, splenomegaly, and hematopoietic panhyperplasia in the bone marrow) also occur in the other MPDs, particularly PV, further obscuring the distinctions between these conditions. It was not until Gunz analyzed 50 cases from the literature plus five of his own that ET became generally accepted as a distinct MPD. In order to establish a diagnosis of ET with confidence, emphasis must be placed upon exclusion of PV, CGL, and IMF/AMM.

Epidemiology

The median age at the time of diagnosis is approximately 60 years; males and females are affected with equal frequency. While ET is even less common than PV, the use of automated platelet counters has facilitated recognition of the condition in asymptomatic patients. The etiology is unknown.

Symptoms and Signs

Published case reports of ET have traditionally emphasized the frequent occurrence of major thromboembolic and hemorrhagic phenomena including thrombosis of the splenic, cerebral, and mesenteric vessels as well as life-threatening gastrointestinal hemorrhage. Thrombosis may develop in either the arterial or venous circulation, and particularly in the microcirculation. Thrombosis of the splenic vasculature may cause splenic atrophy, resulting in characteristic postsplenectomy changes in the peripheral blood and exacerbation of the thrombocytosis.

The PVSG has recently published a review of the clinical and laboratory characteristics (noted at the time of initial presentation) in 37 patients with rigorously defined ET;

this represents the largest prospectively acquired data base on ET yet reported. Non-specific headaches and weakness, bleeding, paresthesias, dizziness, weight loss, and sweating were the commonest manifestations, occurring in more than 20% of patients. In most instances the bleeding was mild, and the distribution was primarily mucocutaneous (epistaxis and ecchymosis). Fever, visual phenomena (scotomata, amaurosis fugax, transient dimming or blurring of vision), peripheral vascular insufficiency (intermittent claudication, digital ischemia), venous thrombosis, angina and/or myocardial infarction, pruritus, and gout were less frequent. Thus although hemorrhage and thrombosis were common in these patients, catastrophic complications (life-threatening hemorrhage, myocardial infarction and stroke) were experienced by only a minority.

The discrepancy between earlier reports and that of the PVSG most probably reflects differences in diagnostic criteria. In the past, thrombohemorrhagic complications were frequently required before a diagnosis of ET was entertained. In contrast, the eligibility requirements of the PVSG are directed primarily at exclusion of the other MPDs (see p. 48). However, the PVSG criteria may have unintentionally excluded patients critically ill with ET because such patients were unable to complete the extensive investigations required prior to institution of therapy.

Splenomegaly is present in approximately 40% of patients. The degree of splenomegaly is usually mild; the spleen rarely extends more than 3 cm below the left costal margin. Hepatomegaly is less frequent. The remainder of the physical examination is usually unremarkable; ecchymoses may be present, but petechiae and purpura are rarely seen.

Differential Diagnosis

Essential thrombocythemia must be distinguished from other chronic MPDs associated with thrombocytosis, from myelodysplastic syndromes associated with thrombocytosis, and from various conditions in which a reactive thrombocytosis occurs (Table 4).

Diagnostic Approach

The following studies are helpful in determining whether or not a patient with thrombocytosis has ET.

Peripheral Blood. The platelet count is always elevated (Fig. 4), usually above 1 000 000/μl, although counts in the range 600 000–1 000 000/μl are still consistent with a diagnosis of ET. The platelet count in other MPDs does not often exceed 1 000 000/μl, and it is even less likely to do so in reactive thrombocytosis. Platelet morphology in ET is frequently abnormal, with bizarre megathrombocytes and abnormally granulated platelets present; circulating megakaryocytic fragments may also be found in the peripheral blood (Fig. 5).

A mild degree of anemia is present in 15%–20% of patients even if iron deficiency due to overt or occult blood loss is excluded. The red cell morphology shows no characteristic changes other than those associated with coincidental iron deficiency. If splenic infarction and atrophy have occurred, Howell-Jolly bodies, Pappenheimer bodies (siderotic granules), acanthocytes, and target cells will be present.

Table 4. Differential diagnosis of thrombocytosis

I.   *Essential thrombocythemia*

II. *Other chronic myeloproliferative disorders*
   A. Polycythemia vera
   B. Chronic granulocytic leukemia
   C. Idiopathic myelofibrosis/agnogenic myeloid metaplasia
   D. Overlap myeloproliferative disorders

III. *Myelodysplastic syndromes associated with thrombocytosis*
   A. 5q-Syndrome
   B. Idiopathic refractory sideroblastic anemia

IV. *Reactive thrombocytosis*
   A. Blood loss and/or iron deficiency
   B. Splenectomy
   C. Hemolytic anemia
   D. Malignancy
   E. Myelophthisis
   F. Chronic inflammatory disorders
   G. Infection
   H. Drug-induced
   I. Rebound from thrombocytopenia
   J. Exercise

Mild leukocytosis is present in approximately 40% of patients, with white cell counts rarely exceeding $50\,000/\mu l$. When leukocytosis is present, it is almost entirely due to a neutrophilia with or without a mild basophilia and/or eosinophilia. Occasional myeloid precursors and nucleated red cells may also be present.

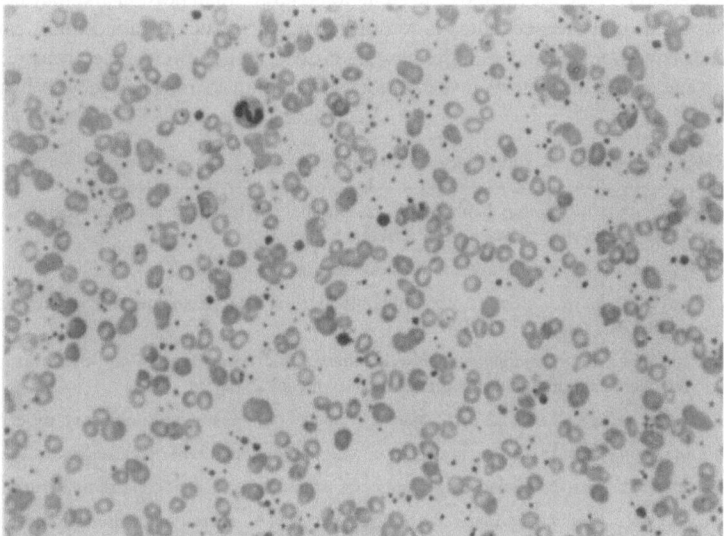

Fig. 4. Peripheral blood in ET showing marked thrombocytosis and several megathrombocytes. ×400

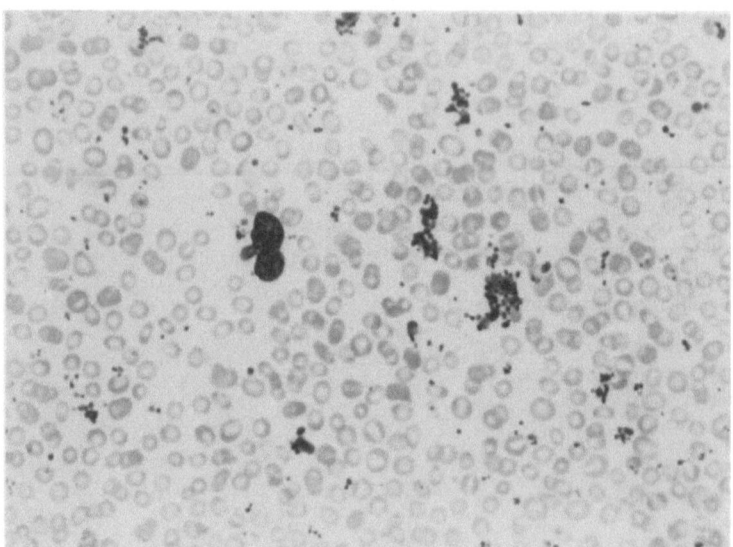

Fig. 5. Peripheral blood in ET showing a megakaryocytic fragment. ×400

Bone Marrow. Aspiration and biopsy of the marrow are primarily helpful in distinguishing between myeloproliferative-related thrombocytosis, myelodysplastic syndromes, and myelophthisic disorders (Table 5). The bone marrow aspirate in ET usually reinforces the peripheral blood findings; massive platelet clumping and megakaryocytic hyperplasia are almost universally present.

As in PV, the megakaryocytes tend to be larger than normal and may be dysplastic in appearance. Increased ploidy is common, and ultrastructural abnormalities of the demarcation membranes and granules have been described; however, electron microscopy is by no means an obligatory investigation. In additon to megakaryocytic hyperplasia, in-

Table 5. Bone marrow appearances in thrombocytosis

Essential thrombocythemia: panhyperplasia; markedly increased megakaryocytes with morphologic abnormalities; iron stores occasionally absent

Polycythemia vera: similar to ET; iron stores almost always absent

Chronic granulocytic leukemia: predominantly myeloid hyperplasia; megakaryocytes may be increased, but smaller size than in ET or PV

Idiopathic myelofibrosis/agnogenic myeloid metaplasia: typically a dry tap; marrow replaced by fibrosis; residual hematopoietic cells predominantly megakaryocytes

Idiopathic refractory sideroblastic anemia: ringed sideroblasts; megaloblastoid dyserythropoiesis

5q-Syndrome: megakaryocytic hyperplasia with hypolobulation of megakaryocytes

Myelophthisis: marrow replaced by tumor cells, granulomas, storage cells, or infarction-induced fibrosis

Other causes of reactive thrombocytosis: megakaryocytes generally increased but morphologically normal; other features variable (see text)

---

creased activity of both erythroid and myeloid elements (trilineage hyperplasia) is present in 75% of patients with ET. When a group of thrombocythemic and polycythemic bone marrows are compared, erythroid hyperplasia is seen to be more marked in PV while megakaryocytic hyperplasia tends to be greater in ET; however, it is extremely difficult to distinguish between these disorders simply on the basis of the morphology observed in an isolated marrow specimen. For instance, the example of a polycythemic marrow in the preceding section (Fig. 2) would also be consistent with a diagnosis of ET.

The likelihood of finding stainable iron in the marrow varies according to the criteria used to define ET (see p. 48). Patients with ET may have iron deficiency due to blood loss; however, if absence of iron deficiency is required for the exclusion of masked PV (this was the case with the series reported by the PVSG), then stainable iron will be present in most cases. If a Prussian blue stain reveals excessive iron stores with numerous ringed sideroblasts, this suggests that the cause of the thrombocytosis is idiopathic refractory sideroblastic anemia rather than ET.

A mild increase in reticulin content is present in approximately 20% of patients at the time of diagnosis. The question of whether or not collagen fibrosis occurs early in the disease is controversial; if collagen fibrosis is a prominent finding, we regard such patients as having IMF/AMM with thrombocytosis. In our experience, patients with only mild fibrosis (i. e., less than one-third of the cross-sectional area of a marrow biopsy) usually have splenomegaly and a leukoerythroblastic reaction as well. We regard this triad of features as characteristic of the cellular phase of IMF/AMM; therefore we classify such cases as IMF/AMM with thrombocytosis rather than ET with marrow fibrosis. This is more than just a nosologic problem, since the median survival of patients with ET is probably at least twice that of patients with IMF/AMM.

Cytogenetics. Nonstimulated metaphases obtained from bone marrow aspirates should be examined for karyotypic abnormalities. Although the majority of patients have normal karyotypes prior to myelosuppressive therapy, karyotypic analysis is important in the search for the Philadelphia chromosome (Ph[1]). This was initially thought to be diagnostic of CGL; more recently it has been detected in several patients whose peripheral blood and bone marrow findings were suggestive of ET. It is not yet clear whether these patients will behave clinically like other patients with ET, or whether they will develop the characteristics of CGL, including acute transformation.

It has been suggested that partial deletion of the long arm of chromosome #21 (21q-) is uniquely associated with ET; but the PVSG, which has accumulated the largest series of rigidly defined ET, has been unable to confirm this. Cytogenetic analysis is also useful for excluding the 5q- syndrome, i. e., deletion of the long arm of chromosome #5, mild thrombocytosis, megakaryocytic hyperplasia with hypolobulation of megakaryocytes, and macrocytic anemia. This condition appears to represent a variant of the refractory anemias which are regarded as myelodysplastic syndromes rather than as MPDs.

Red Blood Cell Mass and Diagnostic Role of Iron Replacement. Since PV and ET share many clinical and hematologic features, determination of the red cell mass is helpful in differentiating these conditions (see p. 38). If iron deficiency is present, the investigation should be deferred until iron stores can be replaced (300 mg ferrous gluconate or sulfate t. i. d), since iron deficiency may mask the erythrocytosis of PV.

Platelet Function. A variety of platelet function abnormalities have been described in the majority of patients with ET. Prolongation of the skin bleeding time, reduced platelet factor 3 activity, reduced platelet adhesion, defective platelet aggregation (particularly with epinephrine), and nucleotide storage pool defects have been most consistently reported. Evidence of platelet hyperaggregability, i. e., spontaneous platelet aggregation and "circulating" platelet aggregates, may also be found. The role of these abnormalities in the genesis of thrombohemorrhagic phenomena is not entirely clear, although several studies have suggested a causal relationship.

Unfortunately, none of these abnormalities are diagnostic of ET; they are often present in patients with IMF/AMM and, to a lesser extent, in patients with the other MPDs. Their major value therefore lies in their ability to differentiate myeloproliferative-related thrombocytosis from reactive thrombocytosis, since the latter is not associated with platelet dysfunction.

Leukocyte Alkaline Phosphatase. The LAP score may be low, normal, or increased. In the series reported by the PVSG, LAP scores ranged from 0 to 171, with a median score of 79. In general, LAP scores tend to be higher in PV than in ET, but there is sufficient overlap to limit the usefulness of this investigation.

Biochemical Findings. Biochemical abnormalities similar to those seen in PV also occur in ET. In addition, pseudohyperkalemia is sometimes present; it is due to excessive release of intracellular potassium from the markedly increased number of platelets during clotting. Simultaneous measurement of plasma and serum potassium will confirm the artifactual nature of the hyperkalemia.

Miscellaneous Investigations. Since thrombocytosis may represent a reactive phenomenon (Table 4), a number of other investigations must be performed before a diagnosis of ET can be reliabl established. The range and intensity of these investigations depend upon the clinical context in which the thrombocytosis was recognized, the available facilities, and the psychological and financial resources of the patient. Most importantly, several stool specimens should be examined to exclude occult bleeding. Various radiologic and endoscopic procedures may be indicated to exclude carcinoma and inflammatory bowel disease; other investigations which may be appropriate include serologic tests for rheumatoid factor and antinuclear antibodies, tissue biopsies for suspected Hodgkin's disease and Wegener's granulomatosis, and microbiologic cultures for tuberculosis and other infections.

PVSG Criteria

The platelet count should be persistently above 600 000/µl, and the marrow should exhibit megakaryocytic hyperplasia. Since ET is not characterized by any unique clinical, hematologic, or histopathologic features, the diagnosis of ET is necessarily one of exclusion. The clinical context of the individual patient determines the investigations required to exclude reactive thrombocytosis. In order to exclude reliably other chronic MPDs, the PVSG has established the following guidelines.

To exclude overt PV, the [51]chromium-labeled red cell mass should not be elevated (males < 36 ml/kg, females < 32 ml/kg). If the red cell mass cannot be determined, then the Hb should be < 13 g/100 ml. To ensure that masked PV has not been overlooked, stainable iron should be demonstrable in the marrow. If it is absent, and the clinical situation permits, a 1-month trial of oral iron therapy should be instituted. The Hb should not

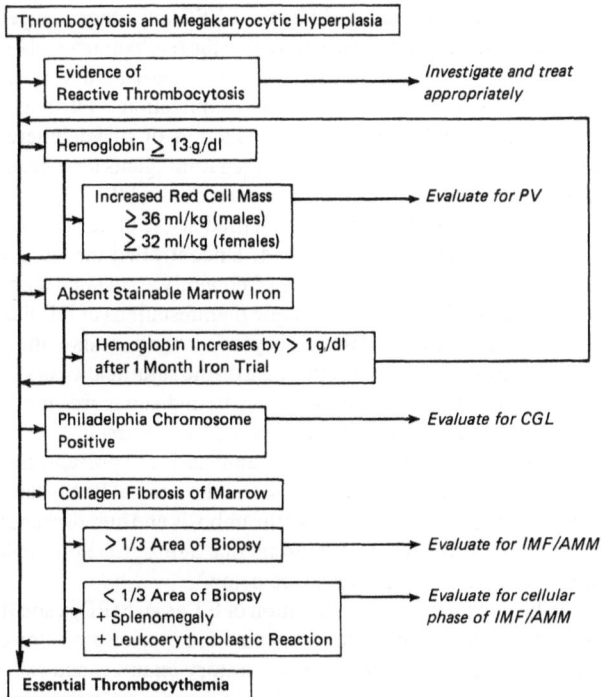

Fig. 6. Schematic approach to the diagnosis of ET [by courtesy of the Association of American Physicians (Iland et al. 1983)]

rise by more than 1 g/100 ml during the period of iron replacement; if the rise in Hb exceeds 1 g/100 ml, then the patient should be reevaluated for evidence of blood loss and/or PV.

To exclude CGL, unstimulated bone marrow metaphases should be examined to ensure that the Ph[1] chromosome is not present.

The extent of collagen fibrosis in a bone marrow biopsy should be determined. Patients with fibrosis involving more than one-third of the cross-sectional area of the biopsy are regarded as having IMF/AMM rather than ET. Patients with the triad of splenomegaly, a leukoerythroblastic reaction in the peripheral blood, and marrow fibrosis involving less than one-third of the cross-sectional area of the biopsy are regarded as having the cellular phase of IMF/AMM. Figure 6 summarizes these guidelines.

Prognosis

Since ET is the least common of the chronic MPDs and has only been widely accepted as a discrete entity for approximately 25 years, little is known about the long-term prognosis of these patients. Earlier reports suggested that ET was associated with major, and sometimes life-threatening, thrombohemorrhagic complications. However, in many of these reports the presence of such complications was required in order to establish the diagnosis.

49

More recent data collected by the PVSG and others suggest that the prognosis is not necessarily so grave, and we believe that the median survival of patients with ET is at least as long as that of patients with PV. Some patients tolerate markedly elevated platelet counts for many years without any complications. Furthermore, in patients with life-threatening complications the introduction of plateletpheresis has brought dramatic responses. Similarly, platelet antiaggregating agents have been shown to reverse incipient gangrene in patients with limb ischemia due to ET.

Unfortunately, the factors which predispose to thrombosis and hemorrhage have not as yet been satisfactorily identified. Uncontrolled thrombocytosis and the presence of platelet dysfunction have been most frequently associated with increased risk. In a recently published review of the neurologic manifestations of ET, the PVSG presented evidence of the role of uncontrolled thrombocytosis in the genesis of these complications. However, the literature contains conflicting data on the significance of such risk factors. For this reason the role of chronic myelosuppressive and antiaggregating therapy in the prophylaxis of thrombosis and hemorrhage remains controversial.

When underlying disorders of hemostasis are present, trauma of any sort (including surgery) imposes additional stresses on the normal hemostatic defenses. ET is no exception, and the risk of perioperative thrombosis and hemorrhage is greatly increased for patients with ET. It is vitally important that appropriate prophylactic measures be taken to minimize such complications (see below).

In keeping with the classification of ET as an MPD, a small proportion of patients undergo transitions to post-thrombocythemic myelofibrosis/myeloid metaplasia and acute leukemia. The clinical features, laboratory features, and survival experience associated with these complications are similar to those seen in the corresponding PV transitional states.

Treatment

The therapeutic approach to ET depends primarily upon the mode of the patient's presentation. Patients with significant thrombotic or hemorrhagic phenomena require swift intervention. On the other hand, if the diagnosis is made fortuitously, less active intervention is indicated.

Major Thrombohemorrhagic Complications

Control of marked thrombocytosis appears to be important in the short-term management of patients with major thrombohemorrhagic complications. Plateletpheresis achieves a dramatic reduction in the platelet count within a matter of hours. Provided the facilities are available, this is the treatment of choice for initial management of patients with clinically significant thromboembolic and hemorrhagic manifestations. Since the thrombocytosis rapidly recurs, myelosuppressive therapy (see below) should be commenced simultaneously, and several more plateletphereses will probably be required before the platelet count is stabilized.

Other Presentations

The appropriate therapy for patients who do not present with major thrombohemorrhagic complications is less well defined. There are three general approaches: myelosuppression, platelet antiaggregant therapy, or no therapy at all. A large-scale randomized trial which allocates patients to one of these three alternatives would be required before definitive statements could be made about the optimal long-term therapy of ET. Since no such trial has ever been conducted, or for that matter is ever likely to be conducted, the choice of therapy remains in the hands of the individual physician.

In deciding on a particular treatment regimen, the clinician must take a number of factors into account, including the patient's age and childbearing potential, the height of the platelet count, the duration, frequency, and severity of symptoms, and the significance of any premorbid conditions. While we cannot claim that these variables reliably predict thrombohemorrhagic risk, common sense dictates that they should influence treatment planning. A number of simple examples are given below to assist the reader in deciding on a treatment program.

A 24-year-old asymptomatic female with a platelet count of $900\,000/\mu l$ requires no therapy other than regular follow-up. On the other hand, a 67-year-old male with unstable angina and a platelet count of $3\,500\,000/\mu l$ clearly requires active therapy, and we would use a combination of plateletpheresis, myelosuppression, and platelet antiaggregating agents. A 33-year-old male with occasional epistaxis and minor bruising could be managed either with no therapy or with myelosuppression; if his platelet count was in excess of $2\,000\,000/\mu l$ then we would be more inclined to use myelosuppression. If there was more significant bleeding, such as a severe gastrointestinal hemorrhage or hematuria, we would plateletpherese and myelosuppress, but would not use antiaggregating agents. A 40-year-old female with a history of amaurosis fugax who has been symptom-free for several months despite a platelet count of $2\,000\,000/\mu l$ should probably be treated with myelosuppression; however, some clinicians may feel it more appropriate to use antiaggregating agents alone. Finally, a 55-year-old male with fever, night sweats, weight loss, and a platelet count of $1\,500\,000/\mu l$ might benefit from myelosuppression, assuming other causes had been excluded (e. g., tuberculosis, carcinoma).

Myelosuppressive regimens are similar to those used in PV, i. e., ^{32}P, alkylating agents, or hydroxyurea (see p. 41 and Table 3). Interestingly, the PVSG has demonstrated that somewhat higher doses of ^{32}P are required in ET ($2.9\ mCi/m^2$). Adequate control can be expected to take from 2 to 6 weeks. As with PV, if myelosuppression is to be instituted, we advocate the use of hydroxyurea in preference to alkylating agents and ^{32}P, particularly in younger patients.

If platelet function studies can be performed, we would also be guided by them to a certain extent. For instance, if the indications for platelet antiaggregating agents were equivocal, we would be more inclined to use them if platelet function studies demonstrated evidence of hyperaggregability. If antiaggregants are to be used, we recommend aspirin (300 mg daily) ± dipyridamole (50 mg tid).

Surgery

The risks posed by surgery for patients with ET have already been emphasized. If surgery is necessary, then the platelet count should be controlled preoperatively, whenever possible by plateletpheresis and/or myelosuppression. Platelet concentrates should be readily available, and should be given prophylactically if major surgery is contemplated. If prolonged immobilization is likely, consideration should also be given to the use of low dose subcutaneous heparin (5000 units, 2 or 3 times daily) to minimize the risk of venous thromboembolism. Platelet antiaggregating agents may also be of value in preventing arterial thrombosis associated with surgery, but the potential value must be balanced against the risks of combined anticoagulant and antiplatelet therapy. We regard the diagnosis of ET as an absolute contraindication to splenectomy unless the patient has reached the equivalent of the "spent phase of PV", i. e., postthrombocythemic myelofibrosis/myeloid metaplasia. All the precautions listed for splenectomy in IMF/AMM should then be taken (see p. 58).

Adjuvant Therapy

The management of pruritus and the prevention of gout and urate nephropathy are as described for PV.

Transitional Phenomena

The management of postthrombocythemic myelofibrosis/myeloid metaplasia and acute leukemia is as outlined for PV.

Idiopathic Myelofibrosis/Agnogenic Myeloid Metaplasia

The third MPD we will consider is idiopathic myelofibrosis/agnogenic myeloid metaplasia. This condition has also been referred to as myelofibrosis with myeloid metaplasia, myelosclerosis, osteosclerosis, aleukemic myelosis , and chronic erythroblastosis.

Idiopathic myelofibrosis (IMF) and agnogenic myeloid metaplasia (AMM) refer to a group of conditions falling within the spectrum of MPD which are characterized by varying degrees of intramedullary fibrosis and extramedullary hematopoiesis (myeloid metaplasia), together with the findings of a leukoerythroblastic reaction and teardrop poikilocytosis in the peripheral blood. The terms myelofibrosis and myeloid metaplasia emphasize different aspects of the pathophysiologic process, and yet the majority of patients exhibit evidence of both marrow fibrosis and extramedullary hematopoiesis (EMH). In our discussion, therefore, we will refer to idiopathic myelofibrosis and agnogenic myeloid metaplasia as a single entity (IMF/AMM). We will also include those patients with marked EMH and minimal fibrosis. The term "cellular phase of IMF/AMM" is sometimes applied to this combination, but it is not clear whether the minority of patients who exhibit only fibrosis or only EMH have a course and prognosis which differs from the more typical cases.

Like the other chronic MPDs (PV, CGL, and ET), the pathophysiology of IMF/AMM is based on disordered biology of the hematopoietic stem cell. Contrary to earlier views, however, cytogenetic and isoenzyme techniques indicate that the bone marrow fibroblasts are not derived from the abnormal clone of hematopoietic cells. Instead, current evidence suggests that growth factors released from the abnormal megakaryocytes and platelets stimulate fibroblastic activity, thus establishing the reactive nature of the fibrosis.

As its name implies, the etiology of IMF/AMM is unknown in the majority of patients. Ionizing radiation and toxins (such as benzene) have been implicated in the genesis of a small number of cases. A virtually identical syndrome ocurs in up to 20% of patients with PV, during the spent phase, and in a small number of patients with ET. Myelofibrosis may be present initially in some patients with CGL, and a myelofibrotic phase may precede the development of blast transformation in others.

A rapidly progressive and fatal form of marrow fibrosis, known as acute or malignant myelofibrosis, has also been described. Although there is considerable debate about this entity, in most instances it appears to represent a variant of acute leukemia; the primitive cells frequently have the typical ultrastructural characteristics of megakaryoblasts.

Epidemiology

Males are affected slightly more commonly than females. The majority of patients are between 50 and 70 years of age when the diagnosis is established, but onset is frequently several years earlier, reflecting the insidious nature of the disease in its early stages. As many as one-third of patients are asymptomatic at the time of presentation, the clinician being alerted to the diagnosis only by the chance finding of splenomegaly or characteristic abnormalities in the peripheral blood.

Symptoms and Signs

The most frequent symptoms are fatigue, weakness, and dyspnea (related to anemia); early satiety, abdominal fullness, and left hypochondrial pain with or without referred shoulder tip pain (due to splenic pressure or splenic infarction); weight loss, fever, and night sweats (associated with a hypermetabolic state); gout, urate nephropathy, and nephrolithiasis (due to increased nucleoprotein turnover); and angina, myocardial infarction, and congestive cardiac failure (related to accelerated cardiovascular disease). Bleeding occurs in 10%–20% of patients and is predominantly mucocutaneous in distribution (epistaxis, petechiae, ecchymoses). Major gastrointestinal bleeding is not uncommon and may arise from peptic ulcers or esophageal varices. Deafness may occur as a result of osteosclerosis. Bone pain is an infrequent initial symptom. Rarely, masses of extramedullary hematopoietic tissue may cause serious complications by virtue of their size and location (e. g., spinal cord compression).

Physical examination reveals splenomegaly in virtually all cases. Splenic size ranges from being just palpable, early in the disease, to massive enlargement extending down to the left iliac fossa and across the midline. Hepatomegaly is present in approximately 70% of patients, but the hepatic enlargement is not as dramatic unless the disease is far advanced. Marked hepatomegaly occasionally develops soon after splenectomy. Other findings include pallor (if anemia is present), lymphadenopathy (in 10%–20%), petechiae, or ecchymoses. Splenic infarction may be accompanied by a friction rub and a sympathetic left pleural effusion. Jaundice and ascites secondary to hepatic EMH and portal hypertension may occur, particularly when the latter is complicated by thrombosis of the portal vein, the intrahepatic sinusoids, or the hepatic veins (Budd-Chiari syndrome).

Differential Diagnosis

Idiopathic myelofibrosis/agnogenic myeloid metaplasia must be distinguished from other chronic MPDs, and from other conditions associated with marrow fibrosis (Table 6) or prominent splenomegaly. Classic cases of CGL can be recognized by the marked leukocytosis, predominant myeloid hyperplasia in the marrow with little or no fibrosis, presence of the Ph[1] chromosome, reduced or absent LAP score, and absence of significant teardrop poikilocytosis. However, atypical examples of CGL, such as Ph[1]-negative CGL, may be impossible to distinguish from IMF/AMM with leukocytosis and minimal fibrosis (the cellular phase of IMF/AMM), and they may in fact be the same disease. Similarly, myeloid metaplasia developing in the course of PV and ET is virtually indistinguishable from IMF/AMM arising de novo.

Carcinoma metastatic to bone may induce considerable fibrosis and a leukoerythroblastic anemia. Adequate biopsy of the marrow is essential to identify this entity, regardless of whether or not there is an antecedent history of carcinoma.

Granulomatous disorders such as tuberculosis, histoplasmosis, and sarcoidosis can all mimic IMF/AMM, and the diagnostic workup should include investigations specifically directed at excluding these entities (chest X-ray, skin tests, microbiological cultures, etc.), In certain situations a trial of appropriate antimicrobial therapy or corticosteroids may be indicated.

A large heterogeneous group of hematologic malignancies characterized by infiltration of the marrow together with marrow fibrosis may resemble IMF/AMM. This group includes hairy cell leukemia, malignant histiocytosis, and atypical non-Hodgkin's lymphoma; they are sometimes collectively referred to as Duhammel's lymphoid myelofibrosis. Acute leukemia may also be associated with an intense reactive fibrosis (acute myelofibrosis); this is particularly true of the megakaryoblastic variants. Morphology and cytochemistry (esterase, tartrate-resistant acid phosphatase, and myeloperoxidase stains)

Table 6. Differential diagnosis of myelofibrosis

I. *Idiopathic myelofibrosis/agnogenic myeloid metaplasia*

II. *Other chronic myeloproliferative disorders*
   A. Chronic granulocytic leukemia
   B. Polycythemia vera
   C. Essential thrombocythemia
   D. Overlap myeloproliferative disorders

III. *Secondary causes of myelofibrosis*
   A. Metastatic carcinoma
   B. Granulomatous disorders
      1. Sarcoidosis
      2. Tuberculosis
      3. Histoplasmosis
   C. Hematologic malignancies involving bone marrow
      1. Acute leukemia
      2. Hairy cell leukemia
      3. Malignant histiocytosis
      4. Non-Hodgkin's lymphoma

are most helpful in differentiating these conditions. If available, immunologic markers and electron microscopy can also provide additional information about the origin of the neoplastic cells.

Finally, other causes of marked splenomegaly may be confused with IMF/AMM. These include lipid storage diseases, splenic lymphoma, and parasitic infections (malaria and kala-azar). They can be identified by their characteristic morphologic appearance in bone marow, blood, or spleen.

Diagnostic Approach

A variety of hematologic, biochemical, cytochemical, radiologic, and cytogenetic abnormalities are present in IMF/AMM, and these can be used to differentiate IMF/AMM from other MPDs and the various secondary causes of myelofibrosis (Table 6).

Peripheral Blood. A normochromic anemia is commonly present. This is associated with a mild reticulocytosis (less than 5%) and abnormal red cell morphology, i. e., anisocytosis, poikilocytosis with prominent "teardrop" forms, and circulating nucleated red cells (Fig. 7). The anemia results from a combination of bone marrow failure, ineffective erythropoiesis in extramedullary sites, pooling of red cells in the enlarged spleen, mild hemolysis due to hypersplenism, and expansion of the plasma volume associated with splenomegaly (dilutional anemia). Occasionally the anemia is exacerbated by concomitant iron deficiency due to bleeding (with hypochromia and microcytosis) or folate deficiency due to the hyperproliferative state (with megaloblastic macrocytosis). Severe hemolysis, evidenced by marked reticulocytosis and shortened red cell survival, develops in a minority of patients.

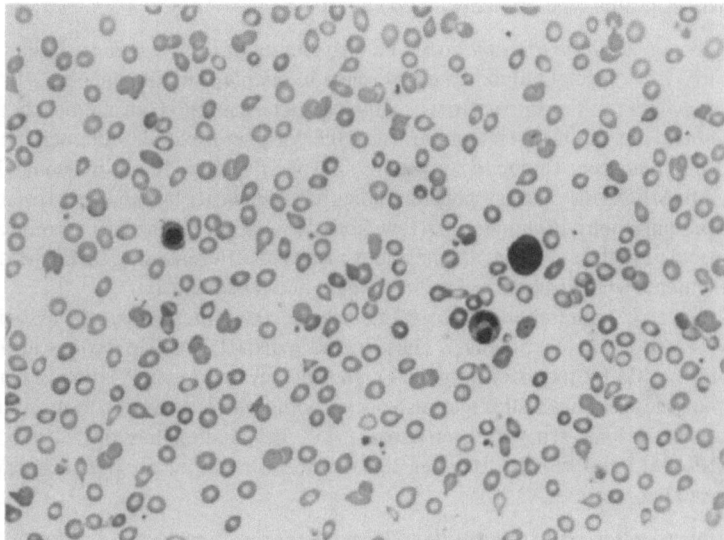

Fig. 7. Peripheral blood in IMF/AMM showing teardrop poikilocytosis; an erythroid and a myeloid precursor are also present. ×400

In approximately half the patients the white cell count is elevated at the time of diagnosis, but it rarely exceeds 50 000/µl. Leukopenia is found in approximately 10%. The differential count reveals mainly mature neutrophilic granulocytes; basophilia and/or eosinophilia may be present. Myeloid precursors are also found in the peripheral blood, and together with the circulating erythroblasts they account for the leukoerythroblastic reaction present in virtually all patients at diagnosis (Fig. 7).

The platelet count may be reduced, normal, or increased; occasionally counts in excess of 1 000 000/µl are seen. As in ET, morphologically abnormal platelets and megakaryocytic fragments are also observed.

Bone Marrow. The bone marow is often impossible to aspirate, resulting in the so-called "dry tap" of myelofibrosis. Needle biopsy is therefore essential, both to demonstrate fibrosis and to exclude certain other diagnoses. Three major patterns of marrow morphology can be identified in the spectrum of IMF/AMM:

1. In some cases the biopsy reveals trilineage hyperplasia without significant collagen fibrosis, either because the fibrosis is patchily distributed or because the degree of fibrosis is truly minimal; the latter situation represents the cellular phase of IMF/AMM. There is usually some increase in reticulin deposition in these cases.
2. The more usual appearance is of prominent collagen and reticulin fibrosis with residual foci of hematopoietic tissue, particularly megakaryocytes.
3. Finally, marked hypocellularity may be present, together with intense fibrosis and osteosclerosis (bony trabeculae occupying more than 30% of the marrow cavity). Residual hematopoietic cells consist mainly of clumps of megakaryocytes.

It has not been established whether the natural history of IMF/AMM involves progression from panhyperplasia to myelofibrosis and osteosclerosis, but since these patients tend to deteriorate clinically and hematologically over time, progressive histologic changes of this type probably do take place.

Leukocyte Alkaline Phosphatase. The distribution of LAP scores is similar to that seen in ET, i. e., normal to moderately elevated in the majority of patients.

Cytogenetics. Since the marrow usually cannot be aspirated, an attempt should be made to obtain unstimulated metaphases from the peripheral blood. Although karyotypic abnormalities occur frequently, most are nonspecific. The Ph[1] chromosome does not occur in IMF/AMM, and cytogenetic studies have primarily been useful in establishing this important point. Prominent marrow fibrosis, absence of the Ph[1] chromosome, and a normal or high LAP score are the major means of differentiating IMF/AMM from CGL in patients who have marked splenomegaly and leukocytosis.

Several nonrandom abnormalities have been described in association with IMF/AMM (and other MPDs). These include partial trisomy of the long arm of chromosome #1 (1q+), monosomy #7 (−7), and trisomy #9 (+9). A combination of the first two of these abnormalities may also occur, with translocation of chromosome #7 to the duplicated long arm of chromosome #1; this finding has only been reported in IMF/AMM and PPMM. Banding studies are essential for the precise identification of these abnormalities.

Demonstration of Extramedullary Hematopoiesis. Fine needle biopsy of an enlarged spleen or liver will reveal trilineage extramedullary hematopoiesis in IMF/AMM, but since the diagnosis can usually be established without this finding, the risk of hemorrhage associated with the procedure outweights the benefit in most circumstances. If demonstration of EMH is considered absolutely necessary, laparoscopic biopsy of the liver via a minilaparotomy is recommended because this combines safety with relative simplicity. Preoperative assessment of hemostatic competence is essential, and platelet transfusions should be admistered prophylactically.

Hemostatic Function. Platelet dysfunction is frequent in IMF/AMM; the abnormalities parallel those previously listed in ET. Since patients with IMF/AMM can experience clinical hemostatic problems in the absence of quantitative platelet abnormalities, it is likely that platelet dysfunction is a significant factor.

In addition, occult disseminated intravascular coagulation (DIC) is sometimes demonstrable. This is manifest by prolongation of the prothrombin time and the thrombin clotting time, elevated levels of fibrin degradation products, reduced levels of factors V and VIII, and increased platelet turnover and activation. A diligent search for DIC should be made whenever surgery is contemplated. The finding of a normal euglobulin lysis time is helpful in differentiating DIC from primary fibrinolysis.

Radiologic Abnormalities. Between 40% and 50% of patients have demonstrable radiologic osteosclerosis. Various patterns have been described, but the most readily recognizable is a diffuse, symmetric increase in bone density involving the axial skeleton (Fig. 8). In most instances this is visible on a chest X-ray. A chest X-ray is also helpful in excluding some secondary causes of marrow fibrosis, such as sarcoidosis and tuberculosis.

Biochemical Findings. Although hyperuricemia and hyperuricosuria are often present, clinical gout is less common. Liver function abnormalities occur, but they are nonspecific and are not useful in establishing the diagnosis or deciding on management. Serum levels

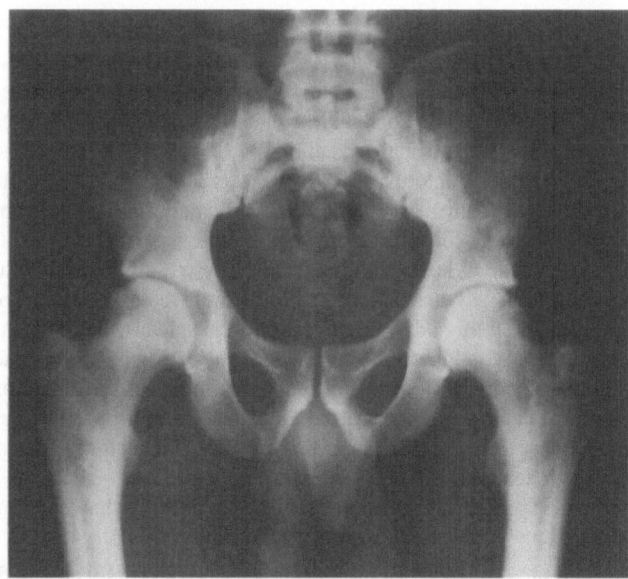

Fig. 8. Radiologic osteosclerosis in a patient with IMF/AMM

of lactate dehydrogenase and histamine are usually elevated. The serum vitamin B_{12} level and the unbound B_{12} binding capacity ($UB_{12}BC$) are normal or mildly elevated.

Prognosis

The survival of patients with IMF/AMM varies considerably; median survival is approximately 5 years from the time of diagnosis. A number of adverse factors at the time of presentation have been identified by retrospective analysis of a large population of patients from the Mayo Clinic. They include the presence of symptoms, significant hepatomegaly, severe anemia, and thrombocytopenia.

The major complications responsible for morbidity and mortality are (a) progressive splenomegaly, with increasing anemia, thrombocytopenia, pressure symptoms, and splenic infarction; (b) degenerative vascular disease resulting in myocardial ischemia, congestive cardiac failure, and cerebral hemorrhage; (c) infections, particularly bacterial pneumonia and tuberculosis; (d) gastrointestinal hemorrhage; (e) acute leukemia, occuring in 5%–10% and phenotypically nonlymphoblastic in most instances; (f) progressive bone pain; (g) urate nephrolithiasis; and (h) progressive ascites and hepatic failure.

Treatment

The primary aim of treatment in IMF/AMM is to improve the quality of life, since there is no evidence that treatment increases survival time. Patients who are asymptomatic probably require no active therapy; early splenectomy has been advocated by some but this remains a controversial option (see below).

Splenomegaly

Splenectomy. Minor to moderate degrees of splenomegaly may cause few symptoms. Acute onset of left hypochondrial pain suggests splenic infarction, and this usually responds to adequate analgesia and rest. Once massive splenomegaly develops, it may cause pressure symptoms while also exacerbating anemia, thrombocytopenia, and leukopenia; the spleen may become chronically painful. These complications constitute the major indications for splenectomy. Splenectomy performed late in the disease is associated with considerable morbidity and mortality, mainly because of the low performance status of the patients (cachexia, advanced cardiovascular disease, severe thrombocytopenia, etc.). It is therefore advisable to remove the spleen when the patient's condition is still satisfactory. Whether splenectomy should be performed prophylactically to delay or prevent these complications is not clear since prospective, randomized studies addressing this question have not been carried out. It has been argued that the liver may become the site of marked myeloid metaplasia soon after splenectomy, thus negating the benefits of early splenectomy.

Once the decision to proceed with splenectomy has been made, it should be performed only under the following circumstances:

1. The surgeon is experienced in the removal of grossly enlarged spleens, which can be a very difficult procedure.

2. The patient has been optimally prepared through adequate preoperative myelosuppression, to minimize postsplenectomy thrombocytosis.
3. A thorough preoperative assessment of the patient's hemostatic competence has been made, including bleeding time, clotting times, evidence of disseminated coagulopathy, and factor assays if appropriate.
4. Adequate platelet and plasma replacement therapy are available.

Prophylactic platelet transfusion should be administered perioperatively, regardless of the preoperative platelet count.

Intraoperative portal venous manometry at the time of planned splenectomy will enable an optimal surgical procedure to be performed. If the portal vein is patent then splenectomy should proceed; if portal hypertension is present, however, then lienorenal or portacaval shunting may be the treatment of choice.

Chemotherapy. Chemotherapy is an alternative to splenectomy particularly for patients who are poor surgical candidates. However, such patients are often exquisitely sensitive to myelosuppression, and dangerous cytopenias may result. The alkylating agents (e. g., busulfan) and hydroxyurea can be used, but therapy with these agents should commence at approximately 25 % of the recommended doses for PV (see Table 3).

Chemotherapy is particularly useful in the perioperative period for the prevention of massive postsplenectomy thrombocytosis. Chemotherapy may also be useful for the small proportion of patients who experience rapid hepatic enlargement soon after splenectomy.

Radiotherapy. Splenic irradiation is another treatment modality that can be used to reduce splenic size, although the duration of the response is usually measured in months. Irradiation should be administered cautiously since there is considerable variation in the responsiveness of patients with IMF/AMM. Patients with acute onset of splenic pain due to splenic infarction may obtain significant and rapid relief from very low doses of splenic irradiation (50–200 rads).

Anemia

As the disease progresses, anemia becomes more severe, and eventually transfusion dependence develops. Nutritional deficiencies (iron, folate, vitamin B_{12}) should be identified and treated appropriately. If ineffective erythropoiesis is the predominant mechanism, androgens occasionally produce an increase in Hb which is sufficient to reduce or even obviate the need for transfusion (e. g., oxymethalone 100–300 mg/day). This therapy should be continued for at least 2–3 months since any effect is usually slow to appear. Hepatic dysfunction is the major side effect. If there is evidence of rapid hemolysis, a trial of corticosteroids is indicated (e. g., prednisone 30–60 mg/day). If the anemia is disabling, particularly if the spleen is grossly enlarged and/or tender, then splenectomy is the treatment of choice (see above).

Thrombocytopenia and Neutropenia

Ineffective thrombopoiesis, trapping of platelets in the enlarged spleen, and increased splenic destruction of platelets are the main causes of thrombocytopenia. Since thrombopoiesis cannot be augmented, splenectomy is the major therapeutic option for severe thrombocytopenia (see above). Splenectomy is also indicated if neutropenia is severe and infections become troublesome. Chemotherapy and splenic irradiation are likely to precipitate problems when used in patients who are already cytopenic, and extreme caution is advised.

Surgery, Adjuvant Therapy, and Acute Leukemia

The approach to surgery, other than splenectomy, is similar to that already outlined for ET (see p. 51). The management of gout, pruritus, and transition to acute leukemia is as outlined for PV (see p. 42).

Acknowledgments. Selected portions of this manuscript have been reproduced by courtesy of the publishers, from the following publications which are currently in press: Current Diagnosis, 7th ed, 1985 (WB Saunders, Philadelphia); Medical Grand Rounds (Plenum, New York); Pathology Update Series (Continuing Professional Education Center, Princeton).

Further Reading

Polycythemia Vera

Dameshek W (1951) Some speculations on the myeloproliferative syndromes. Blood 6: 372–375
Murphy S (1983) Polycythemia vera. In: Williams WJ, Beutler E, Erslev AJ, Lichtman MA (eds) Hematology, 3rd ed. McGraw-Hill, New York, pp 185–196
Silverstein MN (1974) Postpolycythemia myeloid metaplasia. Arch Intern Med 134: 113–115
Weinreb NJ, Shih C-F (1975) Spurious polycythemia. Semin Hematol 12: 397–407
Ellis JT, Peterson P (1979) The bone marrow in polycythemia vera. Pathol Annu 14: 383–403
Berlin NI (1975) Diagnosis and classification of the polycythemias. Semin Hematol 12: 339–351
Loeb V Jr (1975) Treatment of polycythemia vera. Clin Haematol 4: 441–456
Wasserman LR, Balcerzak SP, Berk PD et al. (1981) Influence of therapy on causes of death in polycythemia vera. Trans Assoc Am Physicians 94: 30–38
Rowley JD (1976) The role of cytogenetics in hematology. Blood 48: 1–7

Essential Thrombocythemia

Gunz FW (1960) Hemorrhagic thrombocythemia: a critical review. Blood 15: 706–723
Ozer FL, Truax WE, Miesch DC, Levin WC (1960) Primary hemorrhagic thrombocythemia. Am J Med 28: 807–823
Iland HJ, Laszlo J, Peterson P et al. (1983) Essential thrombocythemia: clinical and laboratory characteristics at presentation. Trans Assoc Am Physicians 96: 165–174
Hoagland HC, Silverstein MN (1978) Primary thrombocythemia in the young patient. Mayo Clin Proc 53: 578–580
Kessler CM, Klein HG, Havlik RJ (1982) Uncontrolled thrombocytosis in chronic myeloproliferative disorders. Br J Haematol 50: 157–167
Jabaily J, Iland HJ, Laszlo J et al. (1983) Neurologic manifestations of essential thrombocythemia. Ann Intern Med 99: 513–518
Murphy S, Rosenthal DS, Weinfeld A et al. (1982) Essential thrombocythemia: response during first year of therapy with melphalan and radioactive phosphorus: a Polycythemia Vera Study Group report. Cancer Treat Rep 66: 1495–1500
Younger J, Umlas J (1978) Rapid reduction of platelet count in essential hemorrhagic thrombocythemia by discontinuous flow plateletpheresis. Am J Med 64: 659–661
Zucker S, Mielke CH (1972) Classification of thrombocytosis based on platelet function tests: correlation with hemorrhagic and thrombotic complications. J Lab Clin Med 80: 385–394
Preston FE, Emmanuel IG, Winfield DA, Malia RG (1974) Essential thrombocythaemia and peripheral gangrene. Br Med J 3: 548–552

Idiopathic Myelofibrosis/Agnogenic Myeloid Metaplasia

Ward HP, Block MH (1971) The natural history of agnogenic myeloid metaplasia (AMM) and a critical evaluation of its relationship with the myeloproliferative syndrome. Medicine 50: 357–420

Rosenthal DS, Moloney WC (1969) Myeloid metaplasia: a study of 98 cases. Postgrad Med 45: 136–142

Laszlo J (1975) Myeloproliferative disorders (MPD): myelofibrosis, myelosclerosis, extramedullary hematopoiesis, undifferentiated MPD and hemorrhagic thrombocythemia. Semin Hematol 12: 409–432

Laszlo J, Huang AT (1977) Diagnosis and management of myeloproliferative disorders. Curr Probl Cancer 2 (1)

Laszlo J (1983) Anemia associated with marrow infiltration. In: Williams WJ, Beutler, E, Erslev AJ, Lichtman MA (eds) Hematology, 3rd ed. McGraw-Hill, New York pp 528–532

Castro-Malaspina H, Moore MAS (1982) Pathophysiological mechanisms operating in the development of myelofibrosis: role of megakaryocytes. Nouv Rev Hematol 24: 221–226

4. Hodgkin's Disease

J. R. Durant

Introduction

The purpose of this essay concerning Hodgkin's disease is to provide a general overview of the disease, to describe the general approach taken at the Fox Chase Cancer Center, and to speculate on future directions which might be taken to improve results. An attempt to present principles is made. Further, it is recognized that the management is complex and often involves sophisticated clinical techniques and equipment, particularly in radiotherapy. In general, if sophisticated staging techniques are not available, surgical approaches will be necessary, and if sophisticated radiotherapy cannot be done, the chemotherapeutic regimens described can be substituted.

The first identification of Hodgkin's disease as a specific entity was made in 1832 by the man after whom the process is named: Thomas Hodgkin. For more than 100 years, the process was considered a malignant disease which had a somewhat variable course but inevitably led to death. Progress in understanding awaited the demonstration that radiotherapy could be given in such a way that some patients were cured, this demonstration being followed by sensible explanations of the reasons for success or failure of the treatment. The belief and then the demonstration that the disease is curable were thus in many respects responsible for the improved understanding that modern oncologists have of this still perplexing process.

Hodgkin's disease is an uncommon malignancy. In the United States less than 8000 cases are expected annually. There is a bimodal incidence by age, with one peak in young adult life and then a gradually increasing incidence with advancing age. In other geographic locations, variations in the pattern seen in the United States occur. For instance, in Japan no peak in early age is reported and, in some undeveloped areas, there is an increased incidence in young males.

Pathologic Clarification

Important progress has been made in developing classifications of the pathologic picture. This progress has been made despite a failure to understand the origin of the malignant Reed-Sternberg cell which characterizes the disease. For many years, the classification of Jackson and Parker was used. This recognized that there were important differences in the behavior of the disease when there were marked deviations from the usual superficial resemblance of the pathologic process to a granuloma. Thus, when the characteristic Reed-Sternberg cells were seen in a very pleomorphic lesion, the designation of sarcoma was made, and, if the lesions had few malignant cells without an obvious granulomatous appearance, it was called "paragranuloma." Sarcomatous lesions has a poor prognosis and paragranulomas a good one. The principles which this classification recognized were real, but it was not a very useful tool for the study of the disease because about 90% of cases fell into the granulomatous category. It remained for Lukes and Butler to refine the observations of Jackson and Parker in order to provide the currently widely used and useful pathologic schema.

No matter what the classification, the diagnosis rests on the identification of the pathognomonic Reed-Sternberg cell, which is classically described as a giant multinucleated cell with prominent single nucleoli which are often eccentrically located within the nucleus. This gives the cell, upon occasion, the so-called "owl eyed" appearance. The disease process replaces the normal architecture of the node or other tissue in which the disease is occasionally found. On the basis of the proportion of these cells to others in the lesion and the degree and type of fibrosis, Hodgkin's disease can be divided into four general types. In one, the least aggressive *lymphocyte predominant* type, Reed-Sternberg cells are rare, and the lesion is made up mostly of surrounding normal, and probably reactive, lymphocytes. At the opposite extreme, Reed-Sternberg cells are abundant and often atypical and provide virtually the entire mass of the lesion. Lymphocytes are few. This type is known appropriately as *lymphocyte depleted* Hodgkin's disease and has the most aggressive natural history. In between there is a variety in which there are quite abundant Reed-Sternberg cells and many lymphocytes. It thus has the features of both of the previously described types and is appropriately called *mixed cellularity* Hodgkin's disease. It has a better natural history than the lymphocyte depleted type but is still considered an aggressive form of the disease. The fourth type is characterized by having the malignant process involving Reed-Sternberg cells and lymphocytes divided by thick bands of collagen which divide the lesion into large nodules. In this variety, the Reed-Sternberg cells often appear to float free in a sea of surrounding lymphocytes and are called "lacunar" cells. This type of Hodgkin's disease is called *nodular sclerosis;* it is more frequent in young women, is associated with late relapse more frequently than the other types, and has a marked tendency to involve the mediastinum.

Pathologists usually have little difficulty in correctly diagnosing Hodgkin's disease, but much experience is required for accurate subclassification into the types described above. Despite this, the classification is useful and can be applied regularly because of the easy availability of slide consultation. Important pathophysiologic, prognostic, and biologic clues of use to the clinician result from accurate subclassification. The lymphocyte predominant type is usually not accompanied by constitutional symptoms and is often localized, where as lymphocyte depleted Hodgkin's disease is often accompanied by constitutional symptoms and is frequently widely disseminated. As noted above, the mediastinum is often the site of nodular sclerosis. Mixed disease is very frequently accompanied by constitutional symptoms and is often disseminated at diagnosis. It is a tribute to progress in therapy that the pathologic classification has little important prognostic impact with modern therapy, being now more a descriptor of the natural history, if untreated.

Other diseases which may be confused with Hodgkin's disease by the pathologist include infectious mononucleosis, where a distinctive clinical picture and diagnostic serology usually preclude the need for a biopsy and thus avoid potential confusion with Hodgkin's disease. Two commonly confused diagnoses are non-Hodgkin's lymphoma and the more recently recognized entity, angioimmunoblastic lymphadenopathy. Occasionally, epileptic patients taking Dilantin will have adenopathy and a drug induced pathologic picture resembling Hodgkin's disease. Most epileptics taking Dilantin who have lymphadenopathy and a pathologic picture of Hodgkin's disease, however, actually do have Hodgkin's disease.

Pathogenesis and Staging

Hodgkin's disease characteristically presents as asymmetric, painless adenopathy. Symptoms characteristic of Hodgkin's disease include unexplained fever, particularly at night, sweating, weight loss, and pruritus. These symptoms, except for pruritus, have unfavorable prognostic significance and are important to the staging system to be described below. Ninety percent of the time, the involved nodes are first found in a lymph node bearing area above the diaphram. Involvement of the tonsils is rare. The nodes tend to be firm and rubbery and may mat together. Other physical findings which may be present include an enlarged spleen and liver. When the disease is far advanced or very aggressive, almost any organ may be involved.

Much of the therapeutic progress made in the disease occurred when it was recognized that although the disease, at first presentation, usually involved supradiaphragmatic node bearing areas, there was often also involvement of the retroperitoneal nodes and the spleen. A further contribution was the demonstration that an enlarged, palpable spleen is not involved by Hodgkin's disease in about 50% of such cases and a normal sized spleen contains Hodgkin's disease as often as 25% of the time. Liver and bone marrow involvement are rare in the absence of splenic involvement. These observations strengthened the basis on which clinical and therapeutic judgments could be made and, therefore, improved results.

Gradually, the true natural history of Hodgkin's disease was outlined, primarily from a series of staging studies. These revealed that contrary to what was long believed, Hodgkin's disease originated as a unifocal process, often in retroperitoneal lymph nodes, and spread in an orderly fashion from one lymph node area to another, progressing from the abdomen to the upper body by invasion of abdominal lymphatics which drained into the thoracic duct. Subsequent observations led to the conclusion that the spleen was more than an enlarged abdominal lymph node. This resulted from its almost essential involvement before a primarily nodal disease became a more widely disseminated one. Subsequently, this notion that extralymphatic disease was always a late manifestation was modified when it was shown that not only did Hodgkin's disease progress in an orderly fashion from one nodal area to another but, like other malignancies, it could also invade locally. Thus, a visceral organ involved by direct spread from an adjacent lymph node did not imply general dissemination. These principles are accounted for in the presently used staging system (Table 1) which, in turn, dictates the staging workup that must be accomplished prior to devising a treatment program.

Table 1. Ann Arbor Staging Classification for Hodgkin's Disease

Stage I	Involvement of a single lymph node region (I) or of a single extralymphatic organ or site (I_E).
Stage II	Involvement of two or more lymph node regions on the same side of the diaphragm (II) or localized involvement of an extralymphatic organ or site and of one or more lymph node regions on the same side of the diaphragm (II_E).
Stage III	Involvement of lymph node regions on both sides of the diaphragm (III) which may also be accompanied by involvement of the spleen (III_S) or by localized involvement of an extralymphatic organ or site (III_E) or both (III_{SE}).
Stage IV	Diffuse or disseminated involvement of one or more extralymphatic organs or tissues, with or without associated lymph node involvement.
A	Asymptomatic
B	Fever, night sweats, loss of 10% or more of body weight.

Symbols for extralymphatic sites: marrow=M; lung=L; liver=H; pleura=P; bone=O; skin=D.

The important historical features in the staging system are the presence of documented, but unexplained, fever greater than 38 °C, with or without accompanying night sweats. Weight loss of more than 10% unexplained by other factors is also important. The presence of these constitutional symptoms has an unfavorable prognostic impact. As already mentioned, Hodgkin's disease is sometimes associated with pruritus, but this has no prognostic importance and does not change the staging. Some patients will have chronic nonproductive cough due to mediastinal or hilar adenopathy.

At Fox Chase, the initial workup includes a careful history to elicit the above described symptoms and physical examination. The physical examination searches carefully for palpably involved enlarged nodes in all of the axially located node bearing areas, particularly the cervical, supraclavicular, axillary, and inguinal areas. As noted before, tonsillar involvement is rare, as is involvement of the popliteal and epitrochlear nodes. Nodes in the mesentery of the abdomen are also usually not involved early in the course of the disease except in lymphocyte depleted Hodgkin's disease. Hepatic and splenic enlargement are carefully sought.

Following completion of the history and physical examination, certain studies are essential. A chest X-ray is always done to determine whether there is mediastinal, hilar or pulmonary involvement. Other studies routinely done include a complete blood count with a platelet count, routine blood chemistry analyses, including the alkaline phosphatase and serum creatinine, and urinalysis. A bone marrow biopsy with a Jamshidi needle is obtained routinely from the posterior iliac crest. Assessment of the abdomen is done with CT scanning. Some institutions still routinely use bipedal lymphangiography, but this is now rarely done in our institution. This combination of studies is usually sufficient to establish the patient's stage according to the Ann Arbor convention, shown in Table 1. If any of these studies are abnormal, additional indicated studies are done to define the extent or the nature of the abnormality. The important question is, however, which patients require laparotomy to establish the true extent of the disease. For instance, if CT scanning and lymphography are not available, an IVP should be done in all cases to rule out ureteral obstruction and then a laparotomy done to establish the stage except when it is obvious that the patient has at least stage IIIB. If radiotherapy is not available staging accuracy regarding abdominal disease is less critical, and chemotherapy can be instituted in the absence of this information.

As improved local radiotherapy gradually improved the outcome for patients with Hodgkin's disease, it became clear that the abdomen was much more frequently involved than was apparent from whatever staging workup was employed at the time. First, the use of lymphangiography demonstrated retroperitoneal involvement not identified by intravenous pyelography. Then, laparotomy revealed splenic involvement not evident by other methods while at the same time it showed that an enlarged spleen did not necessarily mean involvement. Further, nodes not visualized by lymphography could be sampled, particularly those in the hilum of the spleen, the liver, and the epigastrium. The enthusiasm for the improved accuracy of this approach led to its almost routine use in all patients except those who had obviously widely disseminated disease. Gradually, the real value of the procedure was defined as occurring under those circumstances in which unexpected Hodgkin's disease might be found or expected Hodgkin's disease excluded. These circumstances, plus the need to define equivocal findings on other studies or to aid in the delivery of radiotherapy, now provide the indications for laparotomy. Thus, it is no longer necessary to do a laparotomy in an asymptomatic patient whose only abnormality is a node high in the right cervical area, particularly if it is lymphocyte predominant Hodgkin's disease. This quite unusual circumstance is so infrequently associated with inapparent abdominal disease that laparotomy is not necessary. A positive bone marrow biopsy always defines stage IV disease and avoids the need for laparotomy. A clearly positive CT scan in a symptomatic patient also precludes the need for laparotomy but an asymptomatic patient with the same findings requires laparotomy for optimization of radiation therapy planning. Laparotomy and splenectomy should not be undertaken lightly since there is a small but real increase in subsequent pneumococcal sepsis in such patients.

Once the stage of the patient has been established, treatment can be selected. At Fox Chase, we use radiotherapy for stages I-IIIA and chemotherapy for stages IIIB and IV. There are several indications for planned combined therapy involving major radiotherapy and major chemotherapy (see below). Most studies combining these two modalities in all early stage patients in order to improve therapeutic outcome have shown some increase in the remission rate and/or relapse-free survival but no improvement in overall survival. On the other hand, the use of combination chemotherapy in patients who would otherwise be treated only with radiotherapy results in an impressive increase in acute leukemia, the risk of which may be as high as 10% at 10 years. Thus, as stated above, at Fox Chase we routinely use radiotherapy for stages I-IIIA Hodgkin's disease and chemotherapy for stages IIIB and IV.

Radiotherapy for Stages I–IIIA

Principles of radiotherapy include coverage of areas of potential spread beyond demonstrated disease and one use of 3500–4500 rads in between $3^1/_2$ and 5 weeks.

Patients with stage I and IIA disease have a 90% chance of cure with extended field radiotherapy alone. The fields used are carefully shaped with lead blocks and the use of a treatment simulator. Usually, so-called mantle irradiation is given through opposing anterior and posterior parts which include the cervical, supraclavicular, axillary, mediastinal, hilar, and upper para-aortic areas. If there is any mediastinal or hilar involvement, throracic CT scanning is employed in order to define accurately the intrathoracic extent of disease. If this is not done, it is possible to underestimate the extent to which the disease has spread anterolaterally. In the absence of CT, it is unlikely that standard tomography will be a satisfactory substitute, and the therapist will rely on the chest X-ray.

In the usual case of stage I or IIA disease, a laparotomy has confirmed the absence of abdominal involvement as well as removed the spleen. Thus, the abdominal treatment portals need encompass only the para-aortic nodes and the splenic hilum. After the mantle area has been completed, a rest period of 4 weeks is usually given, and the treatment is completed.

Ordinarily, such treatment is well tolerated. Weekly blood counts are obtained and treatment delayed if the WBC falls to below 3000 and restarted when it recovers. As noted, modern radiotherapy departments, including our own, achieve between 90% and 100% complete remissions in stage IA and IIA. Distant relapses and infield recurrences develop in about 20% of cases, but salvage chemotherapy is often successful, with an overall cure rate of 90%. Patients who have IB or IIB disease also receive extended field radiotherapy, but the overall cure rate is less, being about 80%. We treat patients with stage IIIA disease with total nodal irradiation (TNI) and in some institutions TNI is also given for stage IB or IIB disease.

Total nodal irradiation is a complicated program which requires the inclusion of the iliac and inguinal nodes so that the treatment portals abutting against the mantle appear as an anterior and posterior inverted "Y" with an arm extending to the splenic hilum (Fig. 1). Because this program treats much more of the bone marrow than does the extended field approach, treatment delays are more common, and patients experience more fatigue as treatment progresses. This program is very exacting and should be attempted only by experienced radiation oncologists who have linear accelerators available to them. Overall, such patients have a survival at 5 years of about 80%. There is no advantage in routine additional use of chemotherapy in these patients. There are, however, as already men-

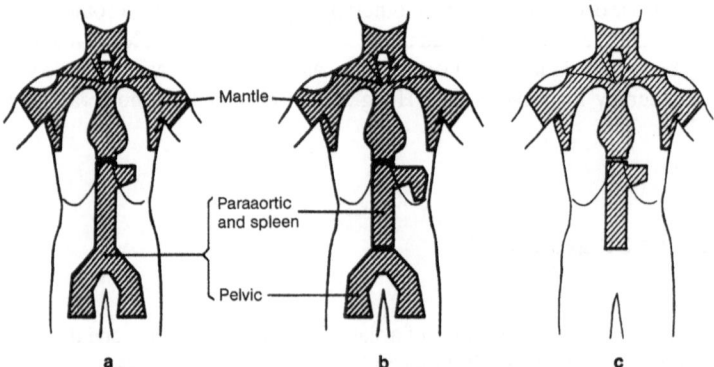

Fig. 1 a–c. Total nodal irradiation fields consisting of a mantle and an inverted 'Y' (**a**) or three fields (**b**). **c** Subtotal nodal irradiation fields after spelenectomy, consisting of a mantle and spade fields

tioned, indications for the combination of TNI and multiple drug chemotherapy. These include those circumstances where there is a greater than 50% probability of death within 5 years. Specific indications include:

1. The presence of extensive mediastinal disease, defined as a mass more than one-third the transverse diameter of the chest in any stage of disease.
2. Stage IIIA with extensive intra-abdominal disease. A cooperative study showed that when there was para-aortic, mesenteric, or iliac node involvement, planned combined modality therapy improved 5-year survival significantly. This study defined the involvement of these areas as stage III_2 and absence of involvement as stage III_1. Another study, at Stanford, showed that there was a significant improvement in survival when there were more than four splenic nodules, if chemotherapy was given in addition to radiotherapy. They could not confirm the results in stage III_2.
3. Multiple direct visceral extensions of disease (multiple sites of true extranodal involvement).

Under all these circumstances, we routinely employ combined modality therapy, believing that extensive disease, as defined by the criteria cited above, is a poor risk factor. This treatment is rigorous and difficult to administer and receive. It should only be used by those experienced in its application.

Because radiotherapy may adversely affect growth centers in bone, children under 15 are treated with particular care, using reduced volumes so as not to compromise growth centers.

Since expensive radiotherapy equipment, particularly linear accelerators and simulators, are essential to the safe, effective administration of radiotherapy when it is relied upon for cure, an important problem arises when such equipment is not readily available and the patient still requires treatment. Under these circumstances, combination chemotherapy as described below may be substituted for radiotherapy.

Chemotherapy for Stages III B and IV

A series of studies done over the years has demonstrated that combination chemotherapy, given intensely for at least 2 months beyond the development of a complete remission, produces complete response rates between 65% and 80%. About 60%–70% of these patients do not relapse. A wide variety of different programs have been used. Most of these are considered to be variations of MOPP (Table 2), developed by DeVita et al. at the NCI. At the Fox Chase center we employ one of these variants (BCVPP), which was developed within the Southeastern Cancer Study Group (SECSG); more recently it has been adopted and extended by the Eastern Cooperative Oncology Group (ECOG). The drugs, doses, and schedule for BCVPP are shown in Table 3. The reason for its use, rather than MOPP, include the lessened incidence of certain toxicities and also a probably improved survival. BCVPP produces significantly less nausea and vomiting, virtually no peripheral neurotoxicity, little platelet suppression, and requires only one visit a month, rather than two, for therapy. In our view, this is sufficient to establish its superiority over MOPP. In addition, however, a recent study reported by the ECOG showed that although BCVPP and

Table 2. Drugs, doses and schedule for MOPP[a]

Nitrogen Mustard (Mustargen)	6 mg/m^2 i. v. days 1 and 8
Vincristine (Oncovin)	1.4 mg/m^2 i. v. days 1 and 8
Procarbazine	100 mg/m^2 p. o. daily × 14 days
Prednisone	40 mg/m^2 p. o. daily × 14 days ONLY 1st and 4th cycle

[a] Cycle repeated every 28 days. Six cycles is standard, but the number should equal either six or two beyond the number required for complete remission, whichever is greater (see text).

Table 3. Drugs, doses and schedule for BCVPP[a]

BCNU	100 mg/m^2 i. v.
Cyclophosphamide	600 mg/m^2 i. v.
Vinblastine	5 mg/m^2 i. v.
Procarbazine	100 mg/m^2 p. o. daily × 10 days
Prednisone	60 mg/m^2 p. o. daily × 10 days

[a] Six cycles is standard, but the number should equal either six or two beyond the number required for complete remission, whichever is greater (see text). Repeat cycle every 28 days.

MOPP produced equivalent complete response rates (75%) in previously untreated patients at 5 years, survival was significantly better for BCVPP (64% vs. 47%). Both regimens are associated with treatment induced leukemias in those surviving up to 10 years. BCNU, however, has the potential to produce up to 1% fatal pulmonary toxicity. No matter what the regimen chosen for initial combination chemotherapy, certain principles should be followed:

1. Treatment should be given at maximally tolerated dose as frequently as possible. Dose adjustment schemes for toxicity are employed regularly. The one for BCVPP is shown in Table 4.
2. Treatment should be given as long as the patient is responding. Most patients will be free of symptoms and signs within 3 months, but some respond more slowly and require continued therapy. a minimum of six cycles is administered and the patient extensively reevaluated. Any questionable areas are subjected to further biopsy. If remission is achieved after 4 months or less, all evidence indicates that therapy can be stopped after six monthly cycles. Maintenance programs of many kinds have been used without benefit. On the other hand, if disease is shrinking but a complete response has not yet been obtained, treatment should continue until two cycles beyond the demonstration that a complete remission has been obtained. BCVPP is probably the preferable therapy when health care facilities are limited because of its ease of administration.

Table 4. BCVPP dose modification[a]

Platelets	WBC		
	< 3000	3000–3999	⩾ 4000
< 75 000	No drugs	No drugs	No drugs
75 000– 99 000	No drugs	50%	50%
⩾ 100 000	No drugs	50%	100%

[a] Discontinue BCNU if unexplained cough and dyspnea appear. Chest X-rays will probably show bilateral hilar and basilar fibrosis. The cyclophosphamide dose should be raised to 1000 mg/m^2.

Salvage Therapy

Although both radiotherapy and chemotherapy are highly successful, some patients fail to achieve complete remission, and others relapse, usually within 5 years. Although a relapse is an unfavorable event in Hodgkin's disease, curative salvage programs exist. If radiotherapy has been the sole prior mode of treatment, it can rarely be used again because the size of the previous dose prevents retreatment if there is an "in field" recurrence. On the other hand, the disease at relapse frequently involves extranodal sites such as the lung, liver, or bone marrow and requires systemic therapy.

Several principles guide selection of salvage chemotherapy for first relapse:

1. Cure is still the goal so that compromises of dose and schedule are made only *after* serious toxicity develops.
2. If relapse has occurred more than a year following completion of prior chemotherapy, reuse of the original chemotherapy regimen is reasonable since complete remission can again be achieved. Pulmonary toxicity is now more likely, and monthly chest X-rays are taken when BCNU is included.
3. If relapse has occurred within a year of completion of therapy or a complete remission has not been obtained, a switch to another regimen is indicated. The usual choice is an adriamycin based combination. Bonnadonna and associates at the National Cancer Institute in Milan, Italy, developed and popularized one of these — ABVD. The drugs, doses, and schedule are shown in Table 5. This regimen contains at least three drugs, adriamycin, bleomycin, and vinblastine, thought not to be cross-resistant with agents in the MOPP program. It has only two agents not found in BCVPP. When MOPP and ABVD have been directly compared, they produce equivalent results, although ABVD produces different toxicities, primarily due to cardiotoxicity from adriamycin and pulmonary toxicity from bleomycin. Both of these are unusual because the total dose of each drug is well below the usual threshold for such toxicity. Suitable monitoring for adriamycin cardiotoxicity is controversial. Therapy should be stopped if arrhytmias develop or if congestive heart failure develops. Similarly, bleomycin should be stopped if cough, dyspnea, and/or basilar rales appear, or if streaky pneumonic infiltrates are seen on the chest X-ray. What to do thereafter is an individual question probably best answered by consultation with someone experienced with these regi-

Table 5. Drugs, doses and schedule for ABVD[a]

Adriamycin	25 mg/m^2 days 1 and 15
Bleomycin	10 mg/m^2 days 1 and 15
Vinblastine	6 mg/m^2 days 1 and 15
DTIC	375 mg/m^2 days 1 and 15

Do not administer a total dose of more than 400 mg/m^2 of adriamycin
Do not administer a total dose of more than 300 mg/m^2 of bleomycin

[a] Six cycles is standard, but the number should equal either six or two beyond the number required for complete remission, whichever is greater (see text). Repeat cycle every 28 days.

mens. Results of ABVD as therapy for relapsing Hodgkin's disease after MOPP therapy are much better in Europe than in the United States; consequently there is controversy as to how much benefit accrues from the ABVD program in patients whose disease is most aggressive. Numerous additional drugs beside those employed in these combinations have been used, but other than VP-16, none seems likely to be very important.

At Fox Chase, we routinely retreat patients relapsing more than a year after initial therapy with their original program and switch to ABVD in those patients relapsing sooner.

Overall results yield 5-year disease-free survival of about 50% for all patients with stage IIIB and IV.

Complications of Treatment

Treatment is not innocuous, and all modalities have both short- and long-term complications, some of which have previously been alluded to. Radiotherapy, particularly if it is not of the total nodal variety, is usually quite well tolerated. Diarrhea, nausea, and vomiting are not usually a problem except with TNI. Most patients receiving mantle therapy will have mild dryness of the mouth and dysphagia, which is occasionally severe. Mild bone marrow toxicity is frequent with extended field radiotherapy, but severe, prolonged suppression is rare. More severe, but usually transient, marrow depression is seen with TNI. Anemia of moderate degree may develop, but transfusion is rarely necessary. Both the lung and the heart are regularly damaged by mantle irradiation. Any lung tissue included in the field develops radiation pneumonitis. This is usually an asymptomatic event noted on interval chest films. About 10% of patients will have a mild nonproductive cough, fever, and dyspnea on exertion; these symptoms can last a few weeks to a few months with spontaneous resolution and no long-term sequelae. No effective treatment is known or necessary. Radiation pericarditis is a potentially more serious problem. About 5% of patients will be found to have an enlarged heart on follow-up chest X-ray. This is usually asymptomatic and due to small or modest amounts of pericardial fluid. Spontaneous resolution without the need for therapeutic intervention is the rule. Some patients will, however, develop cardiac tamponade as a consequence of large amounts of fluid and/or fibrotic constriction of the pericardium. Under these circumstances, partial measures such as pericardiocentesis or creation of a pericardial window almost always fail. Treatment is surgical stripping of the pericardium. This complication is, fortunately, rare, but when it occurs, it usually develops 1–5 years following therapy. A more common complication of mantle radiotherapy is suppression of the thyroid. Biochemical evidence of this, as reflected in elevated TSH levels, occurs in about 50% of patients, and 10%–20% develop frank hypothyroidism which should be treated with thyroid when detected. This is usually a problem from 5 to 10 or more years following completion of therapy. Occasionally, hypothyroidism will be inapparent and associated with pericardial effusion. Thus, it should not be assumed that mantle radiotherapy and radiation pericarditis are responsible for all enlarged hearts seen in these patients.

Complications of chemotherapy are both more frequent and more severe. Nausea and vomiting of variable severity and duration are an almost expected consequence of virtually every chemotherapy program. In the previously mentioned ECOG comparison of MOPP with BCVPP, 84% of MOPP and 64% of BCVPP treated patients had at least some nausea and vomiting. In 17% of those given MOPP, it was considered severe or life threatening as compared with only 3% with BCVPP. Current programs designed to prevent nausea and vomiting have enjoyed only modest success.

Alopecia is almost universal. It is almost always reversible, but many people do not realize that it often involves eyebrows, eyelids, and pubic hair.

Bone marrow suppression should be a goal of therapy and can be coped with using the dose adjustment schedules shown in Table 4. However, it is sometimes severe enough to result in infection, bleeding, and/or the need for transfusion. In the ECOG study cited previously, only 20% had no unusual marrow depression, while about 30% has suppression reported as severe or life threatening. This is a standard complication rate for properly administered programs. In addition, certain chronic toxicities are a regular, although variable, consequence of therapy. Acute leukemia has been previously mentioned in the section cautioning against its use in those likely to be cured with radiotherapy alone. Other second cancers are less common and only questionable secondary to therapy. Other acute toxicities depend upon the drugs involved.

Azoospermia is almost universal in males receiving chemotherapy. With MOPP, it is usually permanent. Other combinations have been less well studied for this effect. The ovary appears more resistant to chemotherapy, and most young women do not become permanently amenorrheic and may have had normal pregnancies after successful chemotherapy. Women in their forties, on the other hand, are more likely to become permanently amenorrheic.

Depressed cellular immunity is an integral part of the disease. It is also a consequence of the therapies used. Almost all patients will have profound anergy following completion of therapy, whether or not a remission develops. Some recovery has been noted to occur slowly in those who never recur but defects are still demonstrable 10 years later. It is not clear whether this is due to the treatment, the disease, or both.

Aseptic necrosis of the head of the femur occurs in some patients as an unusual complication, probably due to the inclusion of steroids in many treatment programs.

Present Studies Testing Ideas for Improving Results

Despite the tremendous advances in therapy over the past 20 years, a small fraction of patients never achieve remission and a sizable minority suffer a recurrence and eventually die of therapeutically resistant disease. Several approaches are being investigated.

1. The use of low dose involved field radiotherapy to previously involved nodes starting about 1 month after induction of complete remission by chemotherapy. Such therapy involves giving about 2500 rads at about 200 rads a day, 5 days a week through multiple individual ports to areas of known disease. It should not be administered until the WBC is above 4000 and the platelet count above 100 000. It may be administered with cobalt or orthovoltage equipment and could be a useful adjunct to chemotherapy in low stage disease when sophisticated radiotherapy equipment and personnel are not available. The Yale group has investigated this in a nonrandomized study for advanced disease and reported a 90% disease-free survival at 5 years for the 84% of patients who developed a complete remission. The ECOG has recently followed up on this observation, comparing the value of such therapy against switching to an adriamycin based combination. Initial results show an advantage to following MOPP with the adriamycin based program rather than low dose involved field RT. Complete remission rates were 76% and 73% respectively, but survival for complete remitters at 5 years was 92% compared to 83%, a difference which was significant (P=0.01).

2. The use of non-cross-resistant combinations. The Milan group pioneered the development of ABVD (Table 5) and compared its use with MOPP and with an alternating combination of ABVD and MOPP. The results indicate superior disease-free survival for the two combinations used in a planned alternating sequence. At 7 years, the survival of MOPP treated patients was 64.8%, compared with 85.4% for the alternating sequence. On the other hand, the SECSG was unable to improve survival by alternating BCVPP with adriamycin, bleomycin, and DTIC when compared with BCVPP alone. The improved results sometimes reported for use of non-cross-resistant combinations remain unestablished, but the Fox Chase Cancer Center is participating in the ECOG study comparing BCVPP vs. BCVPP plus low dose involved field radiation therapy vs. MOPP/ABVD (Fig. 2).

Most recently, an important modification of this approach has been reported by Klimo and Connors and by the Milan group. Klimo and Connors altered MOPP by substituting

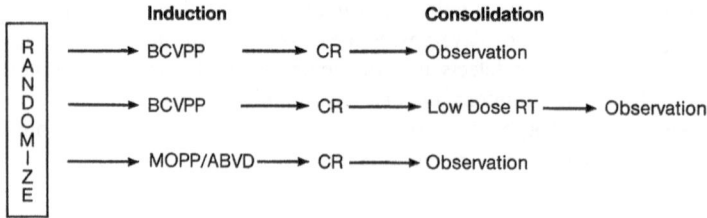

Minimum 8 cycles induction chemotherapy, or CR plus 2 cycles

Fig. 2. Schema of ECOG study 1481. *CR*, complete remission; *RT*, radiotherapy

74

adriamycin, bleomycin, and vinblastine for the second doses of nitrogen mustard, vincristine, and procarbazine in each cycle. Early results of this hybrid indicate complete response rates in previously untreated patients in excess of 90%, with encouraging disease-free survival. Only time will tell whether any of these approaches will improve survival or whether some other fundamentally different strategy will be necessary, such as autologous marow transplantation for certain poor risk categories of patients while they are in remission. The Milan group is currently comparing the alternating combination with a continuous hybrid approach while others are investigating autologous marrow transplantation.

Follow-up

It is important to maintain patients in active follow-up at gradually lengthening intervals. The usual practice in our institution is to see patients monthly for the 1st year, every other month during the 2nd year, every 3 months the 3rd year, every 6 months the 4th year, and annually thereafter. This is important not only for the early detection of relapse but also to monitor for complications. At each visit, a history is taken and a physical examination performed as well as a complete blood count and a chest X-ray. Thyroid function studies are done annually if the neck has been irradiated. Other studies are done as indicated.

It should be realized that not all masses found during follow-up are recurrent disease. Fibrosis and scarring may replace tumors and result in residual, or even recurrent, masses. Recently, impressive thymic enlargement resembling a mediastinal recurrence has been noted in some patients following therapy. If treatment is to be reinstituted, it is usually best to perform another biopsy on the lesion rather than assume a mass is residual or recurrent disease.

Finally, certain infectious diseases may complicate the course of the disease. Most common is reactivation of latent herpes varicella zoster virus. During the first year following therapy, as many as 10% of patients develop shingles, with some cases disseminating. Recently discovered antiviral chemotherapy with adenosine arabinoside (Ara-A) has proven effective in shortening the course of the illness, promoting healing of lesions, and preventing chronic pain. Such an event in the first year after therapy is not associated with an increased chance of relapse, but, thereafter, shingles may be associated with subsequent, or even concurrent, relapse. Other unusual infections which complicate the course of disease are cryptococcosis and cytomegalovirus pneumonia, the latter probably stemming from the use of adrenal steroids in many treatment programs.

Summary

Treatment programs for Hodgkin's disease are increasingly effective. Cure is the goal of therapy in all previously untreated patients and in many who relapse after previously successful therapy. Extended field radiotherapy for stages I to IIB is usually sufficient. TNI is used for stage IIIA. Combination chemotherapy is used for stages IIIB and IV. A combination of TNI and multiple drug chemotherapy is used for specific indications in certain patients with early stage disease. Where sophisticated radiotherapy is not available, combination chemotherapy can be relied upon as the sole treatment program. Successful treatment depends upon accurate pathologic diagnosis and careful staging. Careful follow-up is necessary for early detection of recurrence and quick, effective management of the many complications of therapy. Many new approches to therapy offer the promise of improved results, but there are many unresolved problems in our understanding of Hodgkin's disease.

Further Reading

Bakemeier RF, Anderson JR, Castello W et al. (1984) BCVPP chemotherapy for advanced Hodgkin's disease: evidence for greater duration of complete remission, greater survival, and less toxicity than with a MOPP regimen. Ann Intern Med 101: 447–456

Carbone PP, Kaplan HS, Masshoff K et al. (1971) Report of the committee on Hodgkin's disease staging. Cancer Res 31: 1860–1861

DeVita VT Jr (1982) Principles of chemotherapy. In: DeVita VT Jr, Hellman S, Rosenberg SA (eds) Cancer principles and practice of oncology. Lippincott, Philadelphia, pp 132–155

DeVita VT, Serpick AA, Carbone PP (1970) Combination chemotherapy in the treatment of advanced Hodgkin's disease. Ann Intern Med 73: 891–895

Durant JR, Gams RA, Velz-Garcia E et al. (1978) BCNU, velban, cyclophosphamide, procarbazine, and prednisone (BVCPP) in advanced Hodgkin's disease. Cancer 42: 2101–2110

Lukes RJ, Butler JJ, Hicks ED (1966) Natural history of Hodgkin's disease as related to its pathologic picture. Cancer 19: 317–344

Rosenberg SA (1985) Hodgkin's disease. In: Galabresi P, Schein PS, Rosenberg SA (eds) Medical oncology, basic principles and clinical management of cancer. Macmillan, New York, pp. 457–475

5. Non-Hodgkin's Lymphoma

C. S. Portlock

Introduction

The non-Hodgkin's lymphomas are composed of at least 10 different diseases, according to the U.S. National Cancer Institute Working Formulation for Clinical Usage (see Table 1). This Formulation acts as a "dictionary" of terms to which other classifications, i. e., Rappaport, Lukes-Collins, and WHO, may be correlated. Table 1 provides a cross-correlation of the Working Formulation with the WHO classification.

Table 1. The Working Formulation of the Non-Hodgkin's Lymphomas and the World Health Organization Classification

Working Formulation	WHO
Low grade	
Small lymphocytic (SLL)	Lymphocytic
Follicular, predominantly small cleaved cell (FSCL)	Nodular prolymphocytic
Follicular, mixed small cleaved and large cell (FM)	Nodular, prolymphocytic – lymphoblastic
Intermediate grade	
Follicular, predominantly large cell (FLL)	Nodular, prolymphocytic – lymphoblastic
Diffuse, small cleaved cell (DSCL)	Diffuse prolymphocytic
Diffuse, mixed small and large cell (DML)	Diffuse prolymphocytic – lymphoblastic
Diffuse, large cell (DLL)	Diffuse lymphosarcoma, prolymphocytic-lymphoblastic
High grade	
Large cell, immunoblastic (IBL)	Diffuse lymphosarcoma, immunoblastic
Small noncleaved cell (SNC)	Burkitt's tumor
Lymphoblastic (LBL)	Diffuse lymphosarcoma, lymphoblastic

Each disease category of the Working Formulation has a distinct clinical presentation and prognosis. For the purposes of management, however, it is useful to group the lymphomas into two broad categories: indolent lymphomas, i. e., those diseases which progress slowly and have a long natural history (the low grade lymphomas of the Working Formulation), and aggressive lymphomas, i. e., those diseases which progress rapidly and, if unsuccessfully treated, are soon fatal (the intermediate and high grade lymphomas of the Working Formulation).

It is useful to outline the characteristics of each disease entity before discussing management (Table 2).

Table 2. Pathology and disease characteristics

Malignant lymphoma	Median age	Male: female	Lymph node involvement %		Bone marrow involved %	Median survival (years)
			Local	Generalized		
Low grade						
Small lymphocytic (SLL)	60	1:1	–	100	75	6+
Follicular, small cleaved cell (FSCL)	55	1:1	20	80	50–75	6+
Follicular, mixed small cleaved and large cell (FML)	55	1:1	30–40	60–70	30	5
Intermediate grade						
Follicular, large cell (FLL)	55	2:1	50+	(1)[a]	33	3
Diffuse, small cleaved cell (DSCL)	55	2:1	25	(2)[a]	Common	3
Diffuse, mixed small and large cell (DML)	60	1:1	50	ND	15	3
Diffuse, large cell (DLL)	55	1:1	50	(3)[a]	10	1.5
High grade						
Large cell, immunoblastic (IBL)	50	1.5:1	50+	ND	10	1
Lymphoblastic (LBL)	17	2:1	25	75	100	2
Small, noncleaved cell (SNC)	30	3:1	33	ND	15	NS

[a] Extranodal involvement: (1)=50%; (2)=67%; (3)=frequent.
NS, not specified but 25% disease-free at 5 years.
ND, not determined.

Pathology

Low Grade Lymphomas

1. *Malignant lymphoma, small lymphocytic (SLL).* The median age at diagnosis is approximately 60 years, and this disease is rarely seen below age 30. Males and females are equally affected. Virtually all patients will have generalized lymph node involvement. The bone marrow is also involved in more than 75% of patients. Median survival is at least 6 years.

2. *Malignant lymphoma, follicular, predominantly small cleaved cell (FSCL).* The median age at diagnosis is approximately 55 years, and this disease is rarely seen below age 30. Males and females are equally affected. Approximately 20% of patients will have localized lymph node involvement (stages I and II), and the remainder generalized adenopathy. Bone marrow involvement is documented in 50%–75% of patients. Median survival is at least 6 years.

3. *Malignant lymphoma, follicular, mixed small cleaved and large cell (FML).* The median age at diagnosis is approximately 55 years, and this disease is rarely seen below age 30. Males and females are equally affected. Approximately 30%–40% of patients will have localized lymph node involvement (stages I and II), and the remainder generalized adenopathy. Bone marrow involvement is documented in 30% of patients. Median survival is 5 years.

There are a number of general features of low grade lymphomas, including the following:

— Lymph nodes are rubbery and mobile. They are rarely fixed, and do not have overlying skin infiltration. The nodes may be very bulky but usually are not tender.
— The liver and spleen are frequently involved and may be enlarged. Liver function tests are usually normal, except for the alkaline phosphatase, which may be moderately elevated.
— Other less common sites of disease involvement include pleura, lung, skin, breast, and GI tract. In general, when these sites are involved, biopsy is indicated to determine whether a more aggressive lymphoma is present in these tissues.
— Enlarged lymph nodes may cause lymphedema, ureteral obstruction, and epidural cord compression.
— Sites of disease which are *not* involved by low grade lymphomas include the testes and the central nervous system (meninges or parenchyma).

Intermediate Grade Lymphomas

4. *Malignant lymphoma, follicular, predominantly large cell (FLL).* The median age of diagnosis is 55 years, though FLL may be seen in young adults. There is a 2 : 1 male predominance. At least one-third of patients will have localized lymph node involvement (stages I and II). Extranodal involvement is common in the remainder and the bone marrow is affected in one-third. The median survival is 3 years, with 45% of patients surviving 5 years.

5. *Malignant lymphoma, diffuse, small cleaved cell (DSCL)*. The median age at diagnosis is 55 years, with young adults sometimes being affected. There is a 2 : 1 male predominance. Only 25% of patients have localized lymph node involvement, whereas almost two-thirds have extranodal lymphoma. Bone marrow, liver, and skin are common sites of involvement. The median survival is 3 years, with one-third of patients surviving 5 years.

6. *Malignant lymphoma, diffuse, mixed small and large cell (DML)*. The median age is 60 years with few patients presenting at ages less than 30. The male to female sex ratio is equal. Almost half of all patients will have localized lymphoma (stages I and II) and bone marrow involvement is infrequent (15% of patients). Liver, bone, skin, and GI tract may be involved. Median survival is approximately 3 years, with 35% surviving 5 years.

7. *Malignant lymphoma, diffuse, large cell (DLL)*. The median age at diagnosis is 55 years and this histology is not uncommonly seen in young adults. Males and females are equally effected. Almost half of all patients have localized presentations (stages I and II), and bone marrow involvement is uncommon (10%). Liver, bone, lung, skin, GI tract, testis, and central nervous system are frequent sites of involvement. Median survival is 1.5 years, with 35% surviving 5 years.

High Grade Lymphomas

8. *Malignant lymphoma, large cell, immunoblastic (IBL)*. The median age at diagnosis is 50 years, with young adults being affected. There is a slight (1.5 : 1) male predominance. Over half of all patients will have localized disease (stages I and II). Bone marrow involvement is seen in 10%. Other extranodal sites include liver, GI tract, bone, and skin. The median survival is approximately 1 year with 30% surviving 5 years.

9. *Malignant lymphoma, lymphoblastic (LBL)*. Unlike most other non-Hodgkin's lymphomas, the median age at diagnosis is 17 years, although the disease may be diagnosed in the middle-aged and elderly. There is a 2 : 1 male predominance. At presentation only one-fourth of patients will have apparently localized lymphoma, and bone marrow involvement is the rule. Median survival is 2 years, with approximately 25% surviving 5 years.

10. *Malignant lymphoma, small noncleaved cell (SNC)*. Like LBL, SNC has a young median age at presentation (30 years), and an even more striking male predominance (3 : 1). Approximately one-third of patients will present with apparently localized lymphoma. Bone marrow involvement is uncommon at diagnosis (15%), whereas 25% are alive, disease-free, at 5 years with effective therapy.

There are a number of general features of intermediate and high grade lymphomas, including the following:

— In addition to rubbery, mobile lymph nodes, patients may have hard, fixed lymph node masses with overlying skin infiltration. The masses may even be warm, erythematous, and tender.

— Bulky lymph node masses (>10 cm) are commonly present in the mediastinum, retroperitoneum, and/or mesentery.
— Waldeyer's ring may be involved and such involvement is often associated with extranodal disease of the stomach and/or small bowel.
— The liver and spleen are frequently involved and may be enlarged. Liver dysfunction is more frequently encountered (elevated bilirubin, transaminase, alkaline phosphatase, and lactic dehydrogenase) than with low grade lymphomas.
— Involvement of extranodal sites is common, particularly the GI tract, lung, skin, bone, and meninges. Ovarian, testicular, and renal involvement may be present.
— Enlarged lymph nodes may cause lymphedema, ureteral obstruction, vascular obstruction (particularly superior vena cava obstruction), and epidural cord compression.

Early Detection and Diagnosis

The diagnosis of lymphoma is usually based upon a lymph node biopsy. Ideally, the specimen should be an excisional biopsy of a supraclavicular or axillary lymph node. The cervical and inguinal lymph nodes may be nonspecifically enlarged and pathology may be unrevealing. The management of intrathoracic and abdominal presentations are discussed below.

If available, studies for monoclonality performed on fresh tissue may be of value. Also, touch preps taken from the fresh specimen prior to fixation can provide additional cytologic detail. A lymph node biopsy provides both the architectural pattern (follicular and or diffuse) as well as the cytology. A bone marrow biopsy or needle biopsy of other involved extranodal sites will only provide cytology.

It is not uncommon for patients with aggressive non-Hodgkin's lymphomas to present with massive adenopathy limited to the mediastinum, retroperitoneum, and/or mesen-

Table 3. Ann Arbor Staging Classification

Stage I:	I	A single lymph node region
	I_E	A single extralymphatic site
Stage II:	II	$\geqslant 2$ lymph node region on same side of diaphragm
	II_E	A single extralymphatic site plus lymph node involvement on same side of diaphragm
	II_S	Splenic involvement in addition to lymph nodes on same side of diaphragm
Stage III:	III	Lymph nodes on both sides of diaphragm
	III_E	A single extralymphatic site plus lymph node involvement on both sides of diaphragm
	III_S	Lymph node and splenic disease involving both sides of diaphragm
Stage IV:		Disseminated extralymphatic disease

A: without systemic symptoms
B: with systemic symptoms (unexplained fever, night sweats, and/or weight loss of $\geqslant 10\%$ of body weight)

tery. With thoracic presentations, patients may have acute shortness of breath and/or superior vena cava obstruction, preventing immediate biopsy. Under those circumstances, a short course of irradiation is indicated (less than 750–1000 rads total dose, delivered in 150–200 rad fractions to the obstructing mass), followed by biopsy when the patient is clinically stable.

Massive retroperitoneal or mesenteric tumor requires laparotomy with biopsy. It is usually of value to perform an open biopsy of the liver at the same time, whereas splenectomy is unnecessary. Surgical debulking should be limited to the treatment of intra-abdominal Burkitt's (SNC) lymphoma and to the removal of involved GI tract, where appropriate (surgical management is discussed in greater detail below).

Staging

The Ann Arbor staging system developed for Hodgkin's disease is also used for the non-Hodgkin's lymphomas (see Table 3). Although clinically useful, this staging system has several shortcomings when applied to non-Hodgkin's lymphomas. Such factors as site, bulk of disease, and extent of extranodal involvement are not considered. Moreover, the influence of systemic symptoms on prognosis is much less evident in the non-Hodgkin's lymphomas than in Hodgkin's disease. Nevertheless, in spite of the Ann Arbor system's limitations, thorough staging is a necessity in patient evaluation and management.

Non-invasive studies which are appropriate for all patients with the diagnosis of a non-Hodgkin's lymphoma include:

1. History and physical examination with assessment of systemic symptoms (unexplained fever, night sweats, and weight loss)
2. Complete blood count and platelet count (circulating lymphoma cells may be identified, particularly in histologic specimens from low grade lymphomas); Coomb's test if anemic
3. Liver function studies
4. Renal function studies
5. Chest X-ray, PA and lateral
6. Radiologic evaluation of the abdomen:
   a) Computerized tomography can identify enlarged nodes present in the retroperitoneum and mesentery as well as assess ureteral displacement or obstruction.
   b) An intravenous pyelogram may reveal symptomatic ureteral deviation or obstruction, but it does not adequately assess the presence or absence of adenopathy.
   c) Ultrasound may identify hydronephrosis and large retroperitoneal and/or mesenteric masses.
   d) Lymphography will opacify retroperitoneal but not mesenteric lymph nodes and may be a good indicator of disease, particularly in small retroperitoneal lymph nodes.

In practical treatment planning, the most valuable abdominal study is computerized tomography, and the least valuable, lymphography. The major question to be answered by these studies is: is there *threatening* abdominal tumor which will alter treatment planning?

Other studies which may be of value in limited circumstances include:

1. Serum immunoglobulins in low grade lymphomas
2. Bone scan and X-rays in patients complaining of bony pain
3. Upper gastrointestinal series in patients with gastrointestinal complaints, or in patients with Waldeyer's ring involvement
4. Gallium scan in SNC (Burkitt's) lymphoma
5. Cytologic examination of the cerebrospinal fluid in all patients with LBL and SNC lymphomas, and in all patients with intermediate and high grade lymphomas and positive bone marrow examination
6. Computerized tomography or full lung tomography in patients with thoracic disease.

The clinical stage is determined by these noninvasive studies. Approximately 50%–75% of patients with histologically indolent lymphomas will have clinical stage III disease, less than 10% will be stage I or IV, and the remainder will be stage II. Of patients with histologically aggressive lymphomas, approximately 15% will be clinical stage I, 30% stage II, 30% stage III, and 20% stage IV.

While the clinical stage provides useful information about disease extent, it does not assess bone marrow involvement. Positive biopsies may be present in more than 50% of patients with histologially indolent lymphomas and in as many as 30%–50% of those with histologically aggressive lymphomas. Consequently, all patients with non-Hodgkin's lymphomas should have an iliac crest bone marrow aspirate and biopsy. Among lymphomas with high frequencies of involvement, i. e., histologically indolent lymphomas, bilateral biopsies will increase the yield significantly.

Other invasive methods of assessing extranodal disease extent are usually not warranted. Laparotomy is only indicated in those patients in whom a diagnosis of lymphoma must be made on intra-abdominal tumor or when gastrointestinal or bulky tumor is removed prior to treatment. Staging laparotomy as done for Hodgkin's disease is rarely, if ever, indicated.

Treatment Planning

The treatment approach for patients with non-Hodgkin's lymphomas depends upon such factors as histology, stage, sites of disease, and thoroughness of initial staging, as well as the goals and effectiveness of therapy. Standard approaches are outlined in Table 4.

Indolent Lymphomas

Stage I or II

As described earlier, the indolent lymphomas rarely present as stage I or II disease after complete pathologic staging: SLL, 10%; FSCL, 25%; FML, 30%. However, if the ab-

Table 4. Standard approaches to therapy

1. *Indolent lymphomas*	
Stages I and II	Regional field irradiation
Stages III and IV	Deferred initial therapy
	Single alkylating agent chemotherapy
	Combination chemotherapy
	Local field irradiation
2. *Aggressive lymphomas*	
Stage I	Regional field irradiation
Stages I–IV	Combination chemotherapy with or without involved field irradiation
	Central nervous system prophylaxis, as indicated

dominal assessment has not been complete, then intra-abdominal tumor may be overlooked and the frequency of apparently localized disease will increase.

It has been clearly demonstrated that regional irradiation can control pathologic stage I or II disease. As many as 75 % of such patients may remain disease-free at 10 years after receiving extended field treatment with 3500–4400 rads. Patients eligible for such a radiation therapy approach would be primarily those with peripheral lymph node presentations, i. e., cervical, supraclavicular, axillary, and inguinal. Abdominal masses usually require extensive abdominal ports and thoracic presentations are rare. Radiation therapy technique is discussed below.

In summary, if a patient with low grade lymphoma presents with apparently localized disease (stage I or II) on one side of the diaphragm, involving peripheral lymph nodes, then regional radiation therapy is the treatment of choice. This recommendation assumes at least some evaluation of intra-abdominal lymphoma and the absence of bone marrow involvement.

Stage III or IV

The more common presentation of indolent lymphomas is generalized adenopathy and bone marrow involvement in 30%–70% of the patients. In this setting of stage III or IV lymphoma, systemic treatment may achieve complete remission (a complete disappearance of all known tumor) but remission is usually transient (2.5–5 years), and patients are not cured.

Treatment Deferral

It has been demonstrated that as many as one-half of all advanced stage patients may not require treatment at initial diagnosis. This assessment is based upon the observation that, following diagnosis, the median time interval before requiring treatment is approximately 4.5 years. This treatment-free period ranges from a median greater than 8 years for patients with SLL, to 5 years for FSCL, and to 10 months for FML. Since curative therapy is probably not available for patients with advanced indolent lymphomas, deferring treatment following diagnosis becomes attractive as a management strategy — particularly for those with SLL and FSCL.

There are several benefits of deferred treatment, including the following:

1. There may be a prolonged treatment-free period, particularly for SLL and FSCL.
2. There is no exposure to drugs, thus avoiding later drug resistance.
3. Spontaneous tumor regression may be observed.
4. Appropriate systemic treatment may be selected when disease progression occurs.

On the other hand, treatment defferal does involve hazards:

1. There is a need for close follow-up, with visits every 1-3 month.
2. Clinically silent tumors may progress in threatening sites (such as the epidural space).
3. The patient must carry a psychological burden of remaining untreated.
4. The disease may progress in such a manner as to potentially compromise subsequent treatment.
5. The lymphoma may evolve to an aggressive histology which is poorly responsive to therapy.

The decision to defer therapy is based upon the following factors:

1. *Histology:* Only patients with SLL and FSCL are usually eligible. FML progresses more rapidly and usually requires therapy within 1 year of diagnosis.

2. *Stage:* Only patients with generalized adenopathy or those with extranodal lymphoma (usually limited to bone marrow and/or liver) are eligible (stages III and IV). Those with localized adenopathy without bone marrow disease (stages I and II) should receive regional irradiation as discussed above.

3. *Sites and bulk of disease:* A deferred approach is usually appropriate when (a) lymph nodes are only moderately enlarged (< 4 cm), (b) the nodes are not causing marked ureteral deviation and/or obstruction, (c) there is only minimal to moderate splenomegaly (< 5 cm below the left costal margin) without significant blood count abnormality, and (d) extranodal involvement of potentially threatening sites (i. e., lung, bone, epidural or retro-orbital space) is not present.

4. *Pace of disease:* If the lymph nodes have been stable in size, then observation may be reasonable. If the lymphoma has progressed rapidly, then repeat biopsy may be indicated to rule out evolution to a more aggressive histologic form.

5. *Systemic symptoms:* The presence of unexplained fever, night sweats, or weight loss usually requires palliation with the initiation of treatment.

6. *Age:* Deferring treatment is often more suitable in elderly patients.

7. *General medical health:* In some medically ill patients, treatment may be associated with increased risk.

8. *Patient's psychological make-up:* It must be assessed whether the patient can tolerate the burden of not being treated, and whether the patient is reliable for close follow-up.

9. *Ability to assess extent of retroperitoneal lymphoma:* Since ureteral obstruction is a common complication of progressive retroperitoneal disease, it is necessary to have some means of radiologic evaluation of the abdomen if the patient is to be followed without therapy. If it is impossible to evaluate the retroperitoneum by any means, then the conservative approach in such a patient (with stage III or IV disease) would be to initiate systemic chemotherapy.

In summary, treatment deferral is appropriate for approximately half of all patients with advanced indolent lymphomas. The ideal candidate is a middle-aged or elderly patient who is reliable, in whom adenopathy is historically stable or slowly progressive and moderate in size, and in whom pathology reveals SLL or FSCL.

Systemic Treatment

The advanced indolent lymphomas are highly responsive to chemotherapy. Systemic treatment may involve a single agent or drug combination:

1. *Single alkylating agent therapy (pulse chlorambucil or continuous daily chlorambucil or cyclophosphamide):* This is considered the treatment of first choice for progressive SLL and FSCL. Its advantages are its ease of administration and the relative lack of acute side-effects. The major disadvantage is a relatively slow onset of response, more of a problem for continuous daily therapy than pulse chlorambucil.

2. *Combination chemotherapy:* There are two standard drug programs — CVP (cyclophosphamide, vincristine, and prednisone) and C-MOPP (cyclophosphamide, vincristine, procarbazine, and prednisone). Both combinations yield prompt tumor responses with acceptable acute toxicities. Historically, CVP has been used for SLL and FSCL, and C-MOPP for FML.

Either single or multiagent chemotherapy achieves a complete response rate approaching 80%. The median disease-free interval following discontinuance of therapy is approximately 2.5–5 years and may be even longer with C-MOPP in FML. There is no evidence that continuing chemotherapy during remission (maintenance therapy) prolongs remission or survival.

In summary, systemic chemotherapy is indicated in any patient with advanced indolent lymphoma and progressive or threatening disease. Single alkylating agents are usually chosen first for SLL and FSCL whereas C-MOPP is often used first for FML.

Aggressive Lymphomas

The aggressive lymphomas FLL, DSCL, DML, DLL, and IBL are usually managed similarly. LBL and SNC are discussed separately.

Combination chemotherapy has become the treatment of choice in almost all patients with histologically aggressive non-Hodgkin's lymphomas, regardless of stage. The possible exception to this rule is the rare patient with pathologically documented stage I supramediastinal lymphoma. Since staging laparotomies are not performed routinely and are rarely indicated, this presentation is rarely identified.

Unlike in patients with indolent lymphomas, it is *never* appropriate to withhold initial therapy. In fact, it is necessary to expedite evaluation and initiate therapy as rapidly as possible. As mentioned earlier, there may be some circumstances where threatening disease may require emergency irradiation even prior to a pathologic diagnosis. Chemotherapy is not used in this setting since complete staging has not been performed and drug-induced myelosuppression might complicate future surgical biopsy.

Combination Chemotherapy

There are many drug combinations which are effective in the treatment of histologically aggressive lymphomas. The most widely used regimen is CHOP (cyclophosphamide, adriamycin, vincristine, and prednisone). It yields a complete response in 40%–80% of patients, and as many as three-fourths of these complete remissions are durable. In other words, the ability to cure patients with histologically aggressive lymphomas is high, the overall rate approaching 50%–60%.

A second drug combination which is often used in patients with contraindications to adriamycin therapy is MOPP or C-MOPP (M—nitrogen mustard or C—cyclophosphamide, with vincristine, procarbazine, and prednisone). The complete response rate with this combination may be somewhat less than that with CHOP, but as with complete responders to CHOP, remissions are usually durable.

There is no evidence that maintenance chemotherapy prolongs remission duration or survival.

Radiation Therapy

Radiation therapy is *not* a first-line treatment option for patients with histologically aggressive lymphomas. It is an adjunct to effective chemotherapy. There is one setting in which radiation therapy is often considered standard, *following* a successful course of chemotherapy, and that is mediastinal lymphoma. Here, patients achieve complete regression with chemotherapy followed by full dose (usually 3500–5000 rads) irradiation to the involved region.

LBL and SNC

Both LBL and SNC are very rapidly progressive neoplasms that require prompt (in 12–48 h) initiation of treatment. SNC is the only lymphoma which has clearly been shown to benefit from debulking surgery if all known disease can be removed (e. g., a large abdominal mass).

Regardless of stage, all patients should receive combination chemotherapy. In LBL a modified CHOP regimen is often used in which vincristine is given weekly and prednisone is given continuously during induction. In both LBL and SNC, response to chemotherapy may be so dramatic that it leads to a "tumor lysis" syndrome of hyperkalemia, hypocalcemia, hyperphosphatemia, hyperuricemia, and acute renal failure. This should be anticipated, and countered by allopurinol premedication, hydration, and close attention to serum electrolytes and renal function. If possible, dialysis should be available if acute renal failure ensues.

In addition to a modified combination chemotherapy regimen, all patients with LBL and SNC require central nervous system prophylaxis. Although the incidence of meningeal disease is low at diagnosis, subsequent spread to the meninges is common. Many different regimens are available for prophylaxis; however, the most standard is whole brain irradiation (1800–2500 rads) followed by six doses of intrathecal methotrexate (12 mg/m^2, 12 mg total dose, once or twice per week for six doses). This is usually administered as soon as the patient achieves a clinically complete remission (within the first 4 months).

Pretreatment Preparation

Prior to initiating chemotherapy, all pathologic findings must be carefully reviewed, the extent of disease determined, and the goals of therapy (palliative or curative) clearly outlined. Areas of known disease should be carefully measured and recorded so that they can be followed for disease response.

The patient's general medical condition must be assessed and any contraindications to chemotherapy determined (e. g., cardiac disease limiting the use of adriamycin). Prior to the first drug administration it is wise to begin all patients on allopurinol in order to obviate the potential danger of hyperuricemia. This may be discontinued after clinical response is achieved (usually within 3–4 months). With combination drug regimens it is also useful to pretreat patients with antinausea medication, as well as for 24–48 h after their administration, as needed.

All patients should be informed of the potential toxicities of therapy and the need to inform the treating physician promptly if complications develop. For example, fever > 101 °F (38.3 °C) must be evaluated and treated promptly in the setting of drug-induced neutropenia.

Surgery

As previously mentioned, the role of surgery in lymphoma is usually limited to diagnosis. Some specific settings in which surgery plays an important therapeutic role are:

1. *Surgical removal of gastrointestinal lymphoma.* Although lymphoma involving the gastrointestinal tract may be highly responsive to chemotherapy and irradiation, such treatment may lead to perforation, hemorrhage, and infection when responsive tumor invades the full wall thickness. If disease is limited to one or two segments of the GI tract, it is usually reasonable to accomplish surgical removal. However, if disseminated histologically aggressive lymphoma is present, and only one component is GI tract disease, then surgical removal may not be indicated. Rather, low dose (1500–2500 rads) irradiation to the involved segment followed by combination chemotherapy may be more appropriate.

2. *Surgical debulking of SNC lymphoma.* It is recommended that surgical debulking be considered in patients with abdominal SNC lymphoma. This approach may significantly improve the results of subsequent chemotherapy. However, it is only appropriate in patients in whom a large, resectable abdominal mass is present, without other known disease.

3. *Pleural space sclerosis.* Systemic chemotherapy is usually successful in controlling pleural disease. However, uncontrolled pleural effusions may sometimes be the source of significant morbidity when systemic chemotherapy has otherwise been effective. Closed chest tube draining followed by tetracycline sclerosis is frequently of value in these circumstances.

88

Radiotherapy

The role of radiotherapy in the management of patients with non-Hodgkin's lymphomas is generally limited to adjunctive or palliative therapy. Exceptions to that statement are:

1. *Pathologic Stage I and II indolent lymphomas.* As discussed above, excellent long-term disease-free survival can be achieved with involved field or extended field treatment to the affected region. Typical fields would be axillary (involved axilla with or without ipsilateral supraclavicular region), supraclavicular and/or cervical (ipsilateral supraclavicular and cervical regions), or inguinal (involved inguinal with or without ipsilateral iliac region). Total dose is usually 3500–4400 rads delivered in 200–250 rad fractions.

2. *Pathologic stage I, supramediastinal, histologically aggressive lymphomas (FLL, DSCL, DML, DLL, IBL).* Results with high dose irradiation are excellent; however, this requires staging laparatomy to confirm absence of abdominal lymphoma and is usually unwarranted. Typical radiation fields are those described above. Total dose is often higher, 3500–5000 rads, delivered in 200–250 rad fractions.

Adjuvant Radiotherapy

There are some circumstances in which radiotherapy is employed in addition to effective systemic chemotherapy. These include:

1. Irradiation of residual bulk disease following otherwise effective chemotherapy for histologically aggressive lymphomas. Bulky sites such as mediastinum or retroperitoneum may respond less well than peripheral adenopathy. It is often the practice to add irradiation at the conclusion of chemotherapy. Doses employed range from 3500–5000 rads, delivered in 200–250 rad fractions. In general, this approach should be limited to bulky stage I or II mediastinal presentations.

2. Whole brain irradiation for central nervous system prophylaxis. Total dose is 1800–2500 rads in 200 rad fractions.

Palliative Radiotherapy

Local field radiotherapy may provide good palliation for a variety of local problems, such as epidural cord compression, ureteral obstruction, bone pain, and meningeal disease. In general, radiotherapy in these settings is combined with a change of chemotherapy or in addition to chemotherapy. Total dose ranges from 2500–4000 rads, depending upon the intent of treatment and the condition of the patient.

Chemotherapy

Chemotherapy is the mainstay of treatment for almost all non-Hodgkin's lymphoma. As outlined above, it is indicated for progressive stage III and IV histologically indolent lymphomas and for virtually all histologically aggressive presentations. The drugs employed, their drug schedule, and toxicity are as outlined below.

Drugs

Chlorambucil

Chlorambucil is an alkylating agent which is administered by mouth. It may be given as pulse therapy (16 mg/m^2 × 5 days every 28 days) or as continuous daily therapy (0.1–0.2 mg/kg daily). Acute side effects are usually limited to dose-dependent myelosuppression and occasional nausea. Chronic toxicities include bone marrow failure, hemorrhagic cystitis, and increased risk of second neoplasms.

Cyclophosphamide (Cytoxan)

Cyclophosphamide is an alkylating agent which is administered by mouth when given as daily continuous therapy and either orally or intravenously when given as part of a drug combination. Drug dose as continuous daily therapy is 1.5–2.5 mg/kg daily. Acute side effects depend on the dose and route of administration but include nausea, vomiting, alopecia, myelosuppression, and hemorrhagic cystitis. Chronic toxicities may include bone marrow failure and increased risk of second neoplasms.

Hydroxydaunorubicin (Adriamycin)

Adriamycin is an antibiotic which is administered intravenously as part of a drug combination. Acute side-effects include nausea, vomiting, alopecia, myelosuppression, and rarely cardiac arrhythmias. Skin ulceration requiring debridement and skin graft may occur after extravasation. Chronic toxicities include the dose-dependent development of congestive heart failure (the risk increases steeply after 450–500 mg/m^2 and is exaggerated by pre-existing cardiac disease, concurrent mediastinal irradiation or cyclophosphamide administration, and an age greater than 70 years). Since adriamycin is cleared via hepatic metabolism, abnormal liver function requires dose modification. A general rule is: with total bilirubin of 1.2–3 mg/100 ml there should be a 50% reduction; with > 3 mg/100 ml, a 75% reduction.

Vincristine (Oncovin)

Vincristine is a vinca alkaloid administered intravenously as part of a drug combination. The usual dose is 1.4 mg/m^2 per injection, with a maximum of 2 mg per injection. Acute toxicities include skin ulceration with extravasation; paresthesias, numbness, and tingling in a stocking-glove distribution; motor weakness in a peripheral neuropathy distribution; constipation and obstipation; myalgias; and occasionally recurrent laryngeal nerve palsy. Drug dose is modified or discontinued with progressive or marked nervous and motor symptoms. The drug may be restarted at a reduced dosage after symptoms have resolved. Chronic toxicities are persistent numbness and tingling in a stocking-glove distribution. Permanent motor weakness may occur if the drug is not discontinued when weakness first develops.

Procarbazine

Procarbazine is a hydrazine derivative that is taken orally as part of a drug combination. It is a methylhydrazine derivative. The exact mechanism of acute toxicity is uncertain. It may be an atypical alkylating agent or may behave by causing cytotoxicity by auto-oxidation of the methylhydrazine derivative to hydrogen peroxide. The drug is given orally and the usual dose limiting toxicity is hematologic, causing primarily platelet and WBC suppression. Nausea and vomiting are frequent and may be sufficient to require reduction or elimination of the drug. Tolerance of this side effect often develops with continued administration of the drug. CNS symptoms including myalgias, lethargy, drowsiness, paresthesias, and neuropathy and CNS hyperexcitability, including convulsions, are all uncommon but have been reported. Occasional drug dermatities or hyperpigmentation have also been noted. Since procarbazine is a monoamine oxidase inhibitor, it is important to avoid tyramine containing foods.

Prednisone

Prednisone is a corticosteroid whose mechanism of action is unknown but which has some specific lympholytic properties. The major toxicities from short-term use are carbohydrate intolerance, gastrointestinal bleeding, hypertension, osteoporosis, euphoria, depression, and rarely psychosis.

Drug Combinations

CVP

Cyclophosphamide	400 mg/m^2 p. o. d 1-5	
Vincristine	1.4 mg/m^2 i. v. d 1	
Prednisone	100 mg/m^2 p. o. d 1-5	

Repeat every 21–28 days depending upon blood counts

C-MOPP

Cyclophosphamide	650 mg/m^2 i. v. d 1 and d 8
Vincristine	1.4 mg/m^2 i. v. d 1 and d 8
Procarbazine	100 mg/m^2 p. o. d 1–d 10
Prednisone	40 mg/m^2 p. o. d 1–d 14

Repeat every 28–35 days depending upon blood counts

CHOP

Cyclophosphamide	750 mg/m^2 i. v. d 1
Adriamycin	50 mg/m^2 i. v. d 1

| Vincristine | 1.4 mg/m^2 i. v. 1 |
| Prednisone | 100 mg p. o. d 1–d 5 |

Repeat every 21–28 days depending upon blood counts

MOPP

Nitrogen mustard	6 mg/m^2 i. v. d 1 and d 8
Vincristine	1.4 mg/m^2 i. v. d 1 and d 8
Procarbazine	100 mg/m^2 p. o. d 1–d 14
Prednisone	40 mg/m^2 p. o. d 1–d 14

Repeat cycle every 28–35 days depending upon blood counts

Dose Adjustment of MOPP

Dose adjustment of MOPP should be carried out as shown in Table 5.

Table 5. Dose adjustment of MOPP

WBC	Platelets	Dose adjustment
>4000/mm^3	>100 000/mm^3	100% of all drugs
3000–4000	>100 000	100% vincristine, prednisone 50% cyclophosphamide, adriamycin, procarbazine

2000–3000	50 000–100 000	On day 8 only of C-MOPP
		  100% vincristine, prednisone
		  25% cyclophosphamide, procarbazine

<2000	<50 000	No therapy, wait 1 week On day 8 of C-MOPP, withhold all treatment until counts return to normal (2–3 weeks)

Schedule

The goal of all chemotherapy regimens is to induce complete remission. This may require as long as 6 months to 1 year of treatment in patients with indolent lymphomas, and usually less than 6 months in those with histologically aggressive lymphomas.

Prior to each treatment, blood counts are obtained, physical examination is performed, and assessment of disease activity is carried out. As long as the disease is responding adequately, chemotherapy is continued for a minimum of 6 months before pathologic reassessment of complete response. Pathologic restaging includes the repetition of all studies abnormal at treatment initiation, including bone marrow biopsy.

Treatment Duration

If all tests are normal at the 6 month mark, then 2–4 more months of treatment are given. If some of the tests remain abnormal, then there are two options; (a) continue therapy for

2–4 more months or (b) change the drug combination. In general, it is reasonable to continue therapy in patients with indolent lymphoma as long as the response has been good and there is slow but continued improvement. For histologically aggressive lymphomas, it is probably wiser to consider a change in drug treatment if after 6 months a complete response has not been achieved. This usually means moving from CHOP to MOPP.

When a second-line drug regimen is initiated, at least 6 months of therapy should be administered before treatment is discontinued with the patient in complete remission.

Single agent chemotherapy for SLL and FSCL with advanced stage disease should be continued for approximately 6–12 months before restaging. If all tests are normal, then 4 more months of therapy may be given prior to discontinuing treatment.

Failure of Induction Regimen

Indolent Lymphomas

If the patient with SLL and FSCL fails to achieve complete remission with single agent therapy, there are two alternatives: (a) change to a drug combination such as CVP or C-MOPP, or (b) discontinue all therapy and observe. In general, the second option is preferable since the goal of treatment is palliation and patients may remain stable for extended periods.

If the patient with FML fails to achieve complete remission with C-MOPP the same alternatives apply: switch chemotherapy to CHOP or discontinue C-MOPP and observe. In general, it is reasonable to observe, and when disease progression is evident, to initiate CHOP.

As previously mentioned, complete remissions in patients with indolent lymphomas are usually not durable. When the complete responder relapses, it is usually possible to induce a second remission with the same drug regimen or a second drug combination. However, since palliation is the goal of second-line therapy for indolent lymphomas, it is reasonable to observe the patient in relapse (as one would follow selected patients at diagnosis) and to withhold treatment until indicated by disease progression.

Aggressive Lymphomas

Relapse from pathologically documented complete remission is unusual for patients with histologically aggressive lymphomas. The more common problem is the patient who fails to achieve complete remission or who progresses while on first-line therapy. In either case, it is usually reasonable to attempt induction with a second-line drug combination such as MOPP. Unfortunately, it is uncommon for any second-line combination to control the disease permanently.

Locally advanced tumor may sometimes receive palliation from involved field irradiation. When second-line chemotherapy fails, then sequential single agents can be tried, such as VP-16, cisplatin and methotrexate.

Medical Complications of Lymphoma

The lymphomas or their treatment may cause a variety of urgent medical complications. These are briefly outlined below:

1. *Superior vena cava syndrome:* This complication is usually associated with large, aggressive histology lymphomas involving the mediastinum. It may occur at any time during the course of the disease. If present at diagnosis, it may not be possible to obtain tissue until the SVC obstruction is under control. In this circumstance, local field irradiation should be used, limiting the total dose to 750–1000 rads in 150–200 rad fractions, prior to biopsy.

   If the diagnosis is already known by biopsy of other available tissue, then chemotherapy can be used alone or in combination with radiotherapy to control the SVC syndrome.

2. *Ureteral obstruction:* Bulky retroperitoneal adenopathy is usually the cause of ureteral obstruction, although one should also consider an obstructing stone. Combination chemotherapy is often highly effective in rapidly reducing obstructive adenopathy. Radiation therapy can be held in reserve under these circumstances, since the radiation port is often large and may suppress blood counts.

   Another option is the insertion of a ureteral stent or nephrostomy. However, both these options are of much lower priority and should only be considered in patients with unresponsive tumor.

3. *Epidural cord compression:* Bulky retroperitoneal lymphoma may be associated with "dumb bell" protrusions into the epidural space. This complication may occur at any time during the course of the disease. Although epidural lymphoma may respond well to chemotherapy it is standard practice also to give radiation therapy to the involved segment. The dose of irradiation is usually 2500–4000 rads, depending upon the extent of other known disease and the histology.

   Since the neurologic deficit caused by epidural cord compression may progress rapidly and cause permanent neurologic dysfunction, it is important to initiate treatment urgently.

4. *Meningeal lymphomatosis:* Involvement of the meninges is a frequent feature of LBL and SNC as well as of other aggressive lymphomas with bone marrow involvement. Since neurologic dysfunction can progress rapidly, initiation of treatment should proceed rapidly. Several methods are available: Whole brain irradiation (2000–4000 rads in 200 rad fractions) with intrathecal methotrexate is a standard approach. Intrathecal methotrexate (12 mg/m^2 or 12 mg total dose/injection) is given twice per week until the CSF cytology clears and then once per week $\times 4$. This is followed by an indefinite period of maintenance intrathecal methotrexate. More recently, Ommaya reservoir instillation of methotrexate has been used, obviating the need for whole brain irradiation. The dose and schedule of methotrexate are the same as with intrathecal therapy.

5. *Tumor lysis syndrome:* With rapid tumor lysis following combination chemotherapy, patients may develop hyperkalemia, hypocalcemia, hyperphosphatemia, hyperuricemia, and acute renal failure. The complication is most often seen in patients with

bulky SNC or LBL. It should be anticipated by monitoring of serum electrolytes and renal function, pretreatment allopurinol administration, and adequate pre- and post-treatment hydration. If acute renal failure develops, then facilities for dialysis should be available.

Prognosis and End Results

The non-Hodgkin's lymphomas present a challenge to the treating clinician since chemotherapy and radiotherapy can so dramatically alter the course of the disease.

As described above, the median survival of patients with indolent lymphomas is in excess of 5 years. For rare patients with pathologic stage I or II indolent lymphoma regional irradiation may provide prolonged disease-free survival (> 75 % disease-free at 10 years). For the much more common presentation of advanced stage disease, chemotherapy appears highly effective in inducing complete regression (at least 80 % of patients) but remissions are usually not durable. For SLL and FSCL, single alkylating agent or CVP are good treatment options, whereas for FML, C-MOPP is often used, since apparently durable remissions (> 5 years) have been documented in some patients.

The median survival for patients with histologically aggressive lymphomas is rapidly improving as new drug combinations are developed. It is clear that the majority of pathologically documented complete responders are cured of their lymphoma. With the use of combination chemotherapy in stage I and II disease, the ability to cure most early stage patients appears possible. To maximize the cure rate, it is important that pretreatment evaluation be performed rapidly, that chemotherapy be initiated promptly, and that full dose, on schedule drug treatment be administered. If rapid and complete response is not achieved, movement to an effective second-line program may be of value.

Follow-Up

Since the majority of patients with low grade lymphomas are not cured by treatment, close and regular follow-up is necessary. While under treatment, patients are seen at least once per month. After discontinuance of therapy, once every 2–6 months indefinitely.

For patients with histologically aggressive lymphomas, cure may be possible for complete responders. While under treatment, patients are seen at least once or twice per month. After discontinuance of therapy, complete responders are seen every 2–4 months for 2 years, every 6 months for 3 years, and yearly therafter. For partial and non-responders, treatment must continue indefinitely.

Further Reading

Horwich A, Peckham M (1983) 'Bad risk' non-Hodgkin lymphomas. Semin Hematol 20: 35–56
Portlock CS (1983) 'Good risk' non-Hodgkin lymphomas: approaches to management. Semin Hematol 20: 25–34
The Non-Hodgkin's Lymphoma Pathologic Classification Project (1982) National Cancer Institute sponsored study of classifications of non-Hodgkin's lymphomas: summary and description of a working formulation for clinical usage. Cancer 49: 2112–2135
Ziegler JL (1981) Burkitt's lymphoma. N Engl J Med 305: 735

6. Multiple Myeloma

B. Hoogstraten

Introduction

Multiple myeloma is the uncontrolled, malignant proliferation of plasma cells in the bone marrow. In nearly all instances the cells form a single clone, but occasionally the malignant process may have started from two or more cells, and a few patients have been observed in whom a new clone developed during the disease.

The first report of this disease was in a Thomas Alexander McBean, who on a warm day in August, 1844, felt something snap in his chest when he vaulted from an underground cavern. He was treated with bed rest, venesection, and a plaster cast. In the spring of 1845, the pain recurred and despite treatment with "steel and quinine" he became cachetic and died on 1 January 1846 at the age of 45 — 17 months after the first symptom. It was the urine of this patient that was so extensively studied by Dr. Henry Bence Jones, a pathologist at St. George's Hospital, London.

A second patient from Amsterdam was reported by Stokvis, and in 1889, Kahler reported the 8-year history of an obstetrician with the same protein in the urine as found in the urine of Mr. McBean. The name multiple myeloma was first used in 1873 by von Rustizky, a Russian physician working in the laboratory of von Recklinghausen, when he described eight separate tumors in the marrow of a patient. The name multiple myeloma is now in widespread use; however, Kahler's disease and Rustizky's disease may be encountered in German or Russian literature.

Incidence

The annual crude incidence of multiple myeloma varies somewhat in different countries, e. g., 3.4 per 100 000 population in the United States in 1967, and 4.0 in Sweden. An increased incidence has been noted during the past decades and is believed to be due to improved diagnostic technique and better reporting. There is a slight predominance of males over females. The disease mostly affects the older age groups. Whereas in the 1920s the age group 50–60 saw most cases, this has now shifted to the age group 70–80.

Etiology and Pathogenesis

The exact cause of myeloma remains uncertain. Genetic factors may play a minor role since plasma cell dyscrasias have been observed in siblings. Chronic stimulation of the reticuloendothelial system can lead to plasma cell tumors in the laboratory animal, i. e., injection of mineral oil and plastics in BALB/c mice results in plasmacytomas in 60%–70% of the injected mice. The association with chronic infection and amyloidosis in man is well known. Antibody activity of the monoclonal protein has been demonstrated against specific antigens, including streptolysin O, in a few patients. Allergic reactions to vaccines may lead to intense bone marrow plasmacytosis. Viruses have long been suspected as etiologic agents in animal plasma cells dyscrasias, but no firm evidence for this has been shown in man. Humans are living to older ages and the longer chronic exposure to a multiplicity of factors may be responsible for the increasing incidence of the disease in the older age groups.

Clinical Manifestations

Multiple myeloma is a disease with a wide variety of signs and symptoms, as well as organ involvement. The clinically apparent phase of multiple myeloma is probably preceded by an asymptomatic phase which can last for many years, and even decades. During this time it is often impossible to distinguish between the benign and malignant gammapathy, or to state when the benign stage becomes a malignant one. Waldenström has used the term "premyeloma" when a benign monoclonal gammapathy (BMG) has an unusually high value (above 1.0 g/100 ml) of monoclonal globulin. It is impossible to presume that all BMGs ultimately become malignant, yet no patient with multiple myeloma has been reported as having had a normal electrophoretic pattern in the years prior to the diagnosis of myeloma.

Bone Marrow

The diagnosis of multiple myeloma must never be made on the basis of the bone marrow examination alone, since occasionally, reactive plasmacytosis can closely mimic the myeloma. Also, there is no "typical myeloma cell". In some patients the plasma cells look highly atypical and malignant, while in others they appear almost innocent. In general, the marrow contains at least 5%–10% plasma cells, but most patients have a much higher percentage at the time of diagnosis and cells tend to occur in sheets. Some myeloma cells are very large, containing several nuclei. The chromatin is not as coarse as in the normal plasma cell, and the cytoplasm is basophilic, from dark blue to very light.

Attempts to correlate the morphology of the myeloma cells with the type of excreted monoclonal protein have largely failed, although the so-called flame cells are mainly found in patients with IgA myeloma. The erythrocytic elements are usually normoblastic and there is no clear correlation between the degree of marrow plasmacytosis and the degree of anemia.

Protein Abnormalities

Nearly all patients with multiple myeloma have a typical monoclonal serum component and/or light chain protein (Bence Jones). The distribution of these myeloma components in large series is shown in Table 1. The ratio of kappa (K) and lambda (L) light chains in IgG sera is about 2:1, compared with 1:1 in IgA sera. Patients with IgD myeloma are usually heavy Bence Jones protein excretors, and with a few exceptions, these are L chains.

Two or more monoclonal proteins can be found in up to 1% of patients. The development of these bi- or triclonal gammapathies has been observed during the course of the disease in some patients.

IgG myelomas have a greater tendency toward infections, less hypercalcemia, less amyloidosis, and a higher serum monoclonal protein level than the other types. IgA myelomas have more hypercalcemia and also a greater tendency for the IgA protein to form polymers, resulting in more instances of hyperviscosity syndrome.

IgD myelomas occur predominantly in males and in younger age groups. They frequently have lymphadenopathy, hepatosplenomegaly, and amyloidosis. Survival is short. Whereas, the serum electrophoresis often does not show a monoclonal protein, Bence Jones proteinuria is seen in practically all patients. Renal failure and hypercalcemia are prominent in IgD myeloma and contribute to the short survival.

"Light chain disease" tends to have a more malignant course, with more hypercalcemia, renal failure, and amyloidosis than the IgG and IgA classes. Survival is said to be poor, especially for those with L light chain disease; however, this remains a controversial point.

Skeletal Abnormalities

Radiologic evidence of disease is seen in about 80% of patients with multiple myeloma. Characteristic are the round, punched-out lytic lesions without osteoblastic reaction. In some patients, the predominant feature is diffuse osteoporosis. Pathologic fractures are common, especially of ribs, and as compression fractures of vertebrae. The mechanism of the bone resorption is not yet fully understood. The malignant plasma cells produce

Table 1. Distribution of immunoglobulin classes among myeloma proteins

Class	Range %
IgG	50–65
IgA	15–25
IgD	1–2
IgE	Rare
Light chains only	15–25
Nonsecretory	1

increased amount of osteoclast activating factors in vitro. This suggests that the osteolytic lesions and the osteoporosis may be the result of increased osteoclast activity.

A word of warning is needed regarding the isotopic bone scan. This is frequently negative for bone lesions in patients with little or no osteoblastic activity. Therefore, such scans must not be used to detect skeletal lesions in patients suspected of having multiple myeloma.

Other Laboratory Manifestations

Most patients develop a normochromic, normocytic anemia during the course of their disease. Marked rouleau formation can be seen when the proteins are high. Rapid red cell sedimentation is associated with this, but it can be zero in the presence of cryoglobulins. Megaloblastic changes due to true vitamin B_{12} deficiency have been observed.

The leukocyte count is usually normal or somewhat decreased. Plasma cells or myeloma cells appear in the blood of about 15 % of patients and can lead to a plasma cell leukemic picture in a few.

Platelet counts are slightly reduced in most patients, but rarely to level where hemorrhagic manifestations result. When this is seen, there are usually other abnormalities such as increased antithrombin activity, presence of fibrinolysin, decrease in factor VIII, hyperviscosity, or cryoglobulins with an associated vascular defect.

Hypercalcemia ultimately is seen in 15 %–20 % of patients during the course of their disease, but in only 6 %–8 % at the time of diagnosis. Mobilization of calcium from the skeleton in the rapidly growing myeloma and especially bedridden patients can exceed the ability of the kidneys to cope well with all the calcium and results in hypercalcemia. The hypercalcemia is associated with a normal alkaline phosphatase, and usually normal serum phosphate.

Uremia is frequently seen in the myeloma patient. It is usually accepted that Bence Jones protein may damage the renal tubules and eventually impair kidney function. It is rarely reversible unless it is the result of recent hypercalcemia, in which case normalization of the serum calcium may lead to reduction of the azotemia.

Staging

At the time of diagnosis, the total tumor cell burden may range from less than 0.6×10^{12} cells/m^2 to more than 1.2×10^{12} cells/m^2. The labeling index using tritiated thymidine ranges from 0% to 5%. The residual tumor mass during an excellent response after chemotherapy is still large, in excess of 10^{11} cells/m^2. It may reach 2 or 3×10^{12} cells/m^2 at the time of death.

Durie and Salmon have devised a useful clinical staging system (Table 2) which correlates well with patient survival. The system can also be used to develop new clinical trials specifically for the stage of the disease.

Table 2. Myeloma staging system (Durie and Salmon)

Stage	Criteria	Myeloma cell mass

I	All of the following:
	Hemoglobulin >10 g/100 ml
	Calcium normal (≤12 mg/100 ml)
	Normal bone X-ray or solitary
	  bone plasmacytoma only
	Low myeloma protein
	  IgG <5 g/100 ml
	  IgA <3 g/100 ml
	  Urine light chain <4 g/24 h
		$<0.6 \times 10^{12}/m^2$
		(Low)

II	Fits neither Stage I or III	0.6–1.20

III	One or more of the following:
	Hemoglobulin <8.5 g/100 ml
	Calcium >12 mg/100 ml
	Advanced lytic bone lesions
	High myeloma protein
	  IgG >7 g/100 ml
	  IgA >5 g/100 ml
	  Urine light chain >12 g/24 h
		>1.20
		(High)

Subclassification:
A: Normal renal function (creatinine <2.0 mg/100 ml)
B: Abnormal renal function (creatinine ≥2.0 mg/100 ml)

Treatment

In 1983, the Southwest Oncology Group (SWOG) in the USA published the results of a treatment trial which clearly demonstrates the difficulties facing physicians treating multiple myeloma.

In one treatment arm, melphalan and prednisone (MP) were used, while in two other arms, alternating combinations of four drugs were given. Median survival for patients treated with MP was 24 months, as compared with 40 months with alternating combination chemotherapy. Tumor regression of at least 75% was observed in 32% of patients on MP and 54% of patients on the combinations, but the duration of the remission was not affected by the induction regimen used to achieve remission.

Details of these treatment problems are described later in this section. First, the reader will need to ask a few realistic questions:

1. Are all drugs readily available?
2. Does the cost of drugs play a role in selecting the treatment?
3. How often do patients on five- or six-drug combinations have to be seen, compared with those on oral MP?
4. What is the relative toxicity of the two treatment programs?
5. How does an increase in survival of 16 months relate to the answers to questions 2, 3, and 4?

Question 1: Not every country has equal economic access to all drugs. Agents such as adriamycin, Oncovin, and carmustine are expensive and may not be of high priority in areas where infections still far outweigh cancer in importance as a general health care problem. This simple fact often dictates the choice of drug to be used.

Question 2: The cost of drugs can be prohibitive in some countries and in others the government may have to set a quota for the volume of drugs to be imported. But even in well developed countries, both patients and physicians may have to consider the choice of drugs when the patient can ill afford the high price of some medicines.

Question 3: Combinations of five or six drugs given parentally by expert personnel require frequent visits to centers of excellence. Only few such centers may be present in some countries and patients travel long distances under considerable hardship to see a physician. Oral medications which require less frequent visits and give satisfactory results are to be preferred under such circumstances.

Question 4: The multidrug combinations lead to more toxicity than the simple MP. In the SWOG study, life-threatening hematologic toxicity was observed in 15 % of the patients receiving alternating combination therapy, but in only 2 % of those receiving MP. To this must be added the nausea, vomiting, alopecia, and neurotoxicity seen only with the multidrug combinations.

Question 5: The quality of life becomes very important when drug side-effects are added to hardships of travel, long waiting periods, and general conditions which are difficult to imagine unless one has actually seen them. Under those circumstances it is a philosophical question of whether an additional 16 months of living is adequately balanced by the intensity of the treatment.

Single Drug Therapy

Two alkylating agents, melphalan and Cytoxan, produce an objective response in about 50 % of patients with multiple myeloma and are probably equally effective.

Melphalan (Alkeran, L-phenylalamine mustard) can be given in two ways: (a) Continuous regimen — the patient is started on 8–10 mg melphalan per day for 7 days. The daily dose is then reduced to either 2 or 4 mg depending on the results of the blood count. Some clinics use a rest period of 2 weeks following the initial 7-day course of high-dose therapy. Other clinics prefer not to give a high-dose and start with 4 mg daily. (b) Intermittent regimen — a dose of 0.25 mg/kg daily is given for 4 days, usually in conjunction with prednisone 2.0 mg/kg daily, also for 4 days. Courses are repeated every 4 weeks. The response rates with these regimens are about equal.

Cytoxan (cyclophosphamide) can also be given continuously in doses of 50–100 mg/m^2 daily or intermittently, with 0.25 g/m^2 daily for 4 consecutive days to be repeated every 3 weeks. These higher doses require adequate fluid intake of 3–4 liters per day to decrease the risk of hemorrhagic cystitis and bladder fibrosis.

The ease of a small daily dose requiring less frequent clinic visits may make this the preferred schedule in many countries. Although both drugs are alkylating agents, there is no consistent cross-resistance between melphalan and Cytoxan. Satisfactory remissions have been observed with the second agent after the patient becomes more resistant to the first.

In the anemic patient the addition of prednisone leads to a quicker response than either melphalan or Cytoxan alone. Steroids should be discontinued as soon as possible since they tend to increase the osteoporosis.

Prednisone as a single drug is relatively inactive in the treatment of multiple myeloma, although a decrease in myeloma protein can be seen in some patients. Many other agents have been tested, but few have significant effectiveness.

Combination Chemotherapy

Many combinations of drugs have been tried (Table 3). The Southwest Oncology Group has played a leading role in testing various combinations in randomized trials. Criteria for response have changed considerably and recently at least 75 % tumor regression is required before a remission is achieved. This accounts for the 32 % response rate with MP in 1977–1979, compared with 47 % and 41 % in earlier years. However, the median survival of 24 months with MP has remained the same.

Median survival with the three- and four-drug combinations has ranged between 26 and 34 months. The longest survival has been obtained with the sequence of two four-drug combinations, either VMCP+VCAP or VMCP+VBAP. With these alternating combinations, the median survival time was 40 months.

The drug doses in this rather complicated treatment regimen were as follows:

VMCP: vincristine 1.0 mg/m^2; melphalan 6 mg/m^2 p. o. on days 1-4; cyclophosphamide 125 mg/m^2 p. o. on days 1-4; prednisone 60 mg/m^2 p. o. on days 1-4.

Table 3. Combination chemotherapy in multiple myeloma (SWOG studies)

Combination	No. of patients[a]	% responding
MP 1965–68	75	47
MP 1968–70	79	41
MP 1977–79	77	32
MCP	82	40
MAP	73	36
CAP	61	31
MCBP	74	35
VCAP	77	42
VMCP	78	53
VMCP+VCAP	80	58
VMCP+VBAP	80	49

Abbreviations: M, melphalan; P, prednisone; C, cyclophosphamide; A, adriamycin; B, BCNU; V, vincristine
[a] Includes patients with early death.

VCAP: V, C, and P given as in VMCP; doxorubicin 30 mg/m^2 i. v. on day 1.
VBAP: V, A, and P as given in VMCP.
VCAP: Carmustine 30 mg/m^2 i. v. on day 1; VAP as in the other combination.

An equally complicated treatment protocol conducted at the National Cancer Institute consisted of MP for three cycles every 5 weeks, followed by VCAP for five cycles every 3 weeks, then BMP for three cycles every 5 weeks, and, lastly, VCAP every 3 weeks for an additional five cycles. The objective response rate was 60%, but the actuarial median survival was only 26 months.

Radiotherapy

Radiation therapy continues to be helpful in the palliation of persistent painful localized lesions. However, with the advent of successful chemotherapy it is no longer necessary to initiate radiation as first-line treatment, even in patients with severe pain. It is best to start with chemotherapy and reserve radiation for areas of severe pain after at least 2 months of drug treatment. Tumor doses of about 3000–4000 rad in 3–4 weeks are recommended.

Radiation is indicated for long bone lesions which may fracture, for plasma cell tumors causing spinal cord or nerve root compression, and for some extraskeletal plasmacytomas. Surgical decompression for spinal cord compression should be avoided.

Immunotherapy

Immunotherapy has long been considered particularly attractive in multiple myeloma. The overproduction of plasma cells and monoclonal protein would appear to make this disease a prime candidate for immunomodulation with inhibitors of protein synthesis. BCG (bacille Calmette-Guérin) has been given without any success.

Levamisole is a synthetic immunopotentiating agent which increases phagocytosis, stimulates lymphoblast transformation, and increases delayed hypersensitivity. SWOG has tried the addition of levamisole to maintenance chemotherapy in a randomized trial. The difference in survival between the two groups of patients, with or without levamisole, is marginally significant in favor of levamisole. Time will tell whether this difference persists.

Interferons are hormone-like glycoproteins produced by many types of animal cells in response to a wide range of stimuli. They are biologically defined by their ability to inhibit intracellular viral replication. Interferon (IFN) was first described in 1957 by Isaacs and Lindeman. Industrial scale production of IFN is now being accomplished by several companies. IFN trials in myeloma have primarily focused on patients with disease already resistant to chemotherapy. Partial responses have been reported in 15%–30% of patients even when treated de novo. A randomized Scandinavian trial, comparing IFN in 62 patients with intermittent MP in 53 patients, resulted in a median survival of 17 months for IFN and 29 months for chemotherapy. The clinical experience thus far suggests that IFN has activity in multiple myeloma, but insufficient for it to be used as initial treatment.

Special Manifestations

Hypercalcemia. At diagnosis hypercalcemia is present in 6%–8% of patients, and it develops in an additional 10%–20% during the course of the disease. Vomiting, polyuria, polydipsia, and mental confusion are the prominent symptoms. Since patients are usually dehydrated it is necessary to start fluid replacement immediately. This, together with prednisone and chemotherapy, frequently leads to normalization of the serum calcium. When hypercalcemia persists it may be necessary to try mithramycin 25 μg/kg body weight intravenously, over 4–24 h. One or two doses per week are usually sufficient. Caution needs to be taken with patients already on other chemotherapeutic agents, since mithramycin also causes thrombocytopenia.

Solitary Plasmacytoma. Occasionally patients present with a single lytic bone lesion. This can be treated with irradiation only. Although eventually most lesions progress into generalized disease, the survival of these patients is nevertheless much better than that of patients who present with systemic disease.

Renal Failure. Nearly half of patients with multiple myeloma develop renal disease as a result of tubular damage associated with excretion of light chains. However, not all light chains are necessarily nephrotoxic and some patients may excrete more than 1 g light chain protein per day without appreciable dysfunction. Hypercalcemia and the resultant dehydration rapidly lead to uremia and must be treated vigorously.

High fluid intake, prompt treatment of urinary tract infections, and avoidance and treatment of uricemia, as well as antineoplastic therapy, can reduce protein excretion and improve renal function. In severe or acute renal failure, it may be necessary to perform plasmapheresis temporarily.

Hyperviscosity. In 2%–5% of patients with IgA and IgG myeloma, the protein may aggregate, causing a marked increase in serum viscosity. The Sia test is a simple test for recognizing the presence of euglobulins. A drop of serum is added to a tube of distilled water, and if a white precipitate appears, the test is read as positive. Symptoms usually do not appear unless the serum viscosity (relative to water) rises above 4.

Symptoms include easy bruising, epistasis, purpura, retinopathy, retinal hemorrhages, weakness, vertigo, nystagmus, paresis, and coma. The hypervolemia and increased vascular resistance may lead to cardiac failure. Plasmapheresis may be needed in additon to chemotherapy when the symptoms are acute or severe.

Amyloidosis. Primary (immunoglobulin related) amyloidosis is nearly always associated with one or more of the following: marrow plasmacytosis, light chain protein in the urine, and a serum M-protein. Amyloid of this type contains protein consisting of fragments of light chains. L light chains are more likely to form amyloid than K light chains.

Immunoglobulin related amyloid deposits generally are present in the tongue, heart, skeletal muscle, and gastrointestinal tract. However, other organs typically affected in secondary amyloidosis, such as liver, spleen, and kidney, may also be involved.

Patients may present with an enlarged tongue, carpal tunnel syndrome, arrythmias, conduction defects and murmurs, and a wide variety of gastrointestinal symptoms. Kidney involvement leads to damage of the glomerular basement membrane and loss of all proteins in the urine. Chemotherapy may decrease the deposit in a few patients.

Further Reading

Waldenström J (ed) (1970) Multiple myeloma, diagnosis and treatment. Grune and Stratton, New York
Wintrobe MM (ed) (1981) Clinical hematology. Lea Febiger, Philadelphia, pp 1739–1760
Osserman EF (1959) Plasma cell myeloma. N Engl J Med 261: 952–1006
Durie BGM, Salmon SE (1975) A clinical staging system for multiple myeloma. Cancer 36: 842
Salmon SE, Haut A, Bonnet JD, Amare M, Weick JK, Durie BGM, Dixon DO (1983) Alternating combination chemotherapy and levamisole improves survival in multiple myeloma: a Southwest Oncology Group study. J Clin Oncol 1: 453–461
Kirkwood JM, Ernstoff MS (1984) Interferons in the treatment of cancer. J Clin Oncol 2: 336–352

Subject Index